THE GREEN SOLUTION TO BREAST CANCER

THE GREEN SOLUTION TO BREAST CANCER

A Promise for Prevention

KRISTEN ABATSIS MCHENRY, PHD

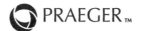 PRAEGER ™

An Imprint of ABC-CLIO, LLC
Santa Barbara, California • Denver, Colorado

Library of Congress Cataloging-in-Publication Data

McHenry, Kristen Abatsis.
 The green solution to breast cancer : a promise for prevention / Kristen Abatsis McHenry PhD.
   pages cm
 Includes bibliographical references and index.
 ISBN 978-1-4408-4034-0 (hardback) – ISBN 978-1-4408-4035-7 (eISBN)
1. Breast–Cancer–United States–Prevention. 2. Breast–Cancer–Environmental aspects–United States. 3. Breast–Cancer–Research. 4. Women–Health and hygiene. I. Title.
RC280.B8M3584   2015
616.99′449—dc23   2015021212

ISBN: 978-1-4408-4034-0
EISBN: 978-1-4408-4035-7

19 18 17 16 15   1 2 3 4 5

This book is also available on the World Wide Web as an eBook.
Visit www.abc-clio.com for details.

Praeger
An Imprint of ABC-CLIO, LLC

ABC-CLIO, LLC
130 Cremona Drive, P.O. Box 1911
Santa Barbara, California 93116-1911

This book is printed on acid-free paper ∞

Manufactured in the United States of America

For Aunt Betty, survivors, and loved ones impacted by breast cancer.
For the one in eight women who will be diagnosed in their lifetime.
This is for you.

Contents

Acknowledgments

I would like to dedicate this book first and foremost to the women who struggle, survive, and have lost their lives to breast cancer. Without their inspiration, hard work, and relentless fight against breast cancer, this work would not have been possible. I thank you for the many women who sat with me and allowed me to listen to their words, thoughts, and feelings on breast cancer. I also want to thank the breast cancer organizations that welcomed me and allowed me to get a closer look at the important advocacy work they are doing.

I am indebted to John Brigham for believing in my research and my abilities as a scholar. I cannot even begin to express how grateful I am for your mentorship and vision. I am always thrilled to see your commitment to interdisciplinary research and I feel incredibly fortunate to have such a skilled and thoughtful mentor. Thank you to Laura Lovett and Jillian Schwedler for your contributions as dissertation committee members, all of who provided valuable suggestions for improving my research and helping craft this research into a book. I owe so much to the faculty of Women's Studies at UMass Dartmouth, for showing me how to let my voice be heard clearly and coherently. Thank you Chris Bobel, Cathy Gardner, Jen Riley, and Banu Subramaniam. Thank you to Allaine Cerwonka for your ongoing mentorship and support. It is because of your words of wisdom and your commitment to Women's Studies that I remain passionate and focused on my feminist journey. I am indebted to Phil Brown, Samantha King, Barbara Ley, and Sabrina McCormick for those of you who were willing to mentor me by commenting on early drafts of this work and offering support as well as inspiration through your own publications. I have been inspired by the research you are doing and thrilled to join this conversation. I would like to show appreciation for my friends who have supported me. Throughout this journey, I have never lacked for words of encouragement. Marita, Julia, Veronica, Yakubu, Inkyoung, Amy, and Moon, you have offered me intellectual support and friendship through the years and for that I thank you.

To my family, I owe you everything. I am here today, accomplishing a dream, because of your sacrifices and determination. It is because of your hard work, help, child care, and endless support that I was physically and emotionally able to complete this. Jason your hope, love, dedication, and confidence in me are what drive me even today. Jason, Connor, Anelie, Mom, and Courtney, I hope this accomplishment has made you proud.

CHAPTER 1

Introduction: The Breast Cancer Movement in the United States

In 1964, the lifetime risk of breast cancer was 1 in 20. In 1984, the lifetime risk of breast cancer for women was 1 in 14. According to the National Cancer Institute, today that risk is 1 in 8. A woman born today has more chance of being diagnosed with breast cancer than in 1964. In the United States, a woman is diagnosed with breast cancer every two minutes (American Cancer Society 2014). This is an alarming pattern of increased risk, and indicates we are not winning the war on cancer. Despite the breast cancer movement's successful ability to increase awareness for early detection and treatment, we still understand very little about the causes of cancer. According to the California Breast Cancer Research Program, 50–70% of women with breast cancer have no known risk factors (CBCRP 2007). Although the breast cancer movement in the United States has quite successfully raised awareness of lifestyle risk factors for breast cancer, increased the visibility of the disease through pink ribbons, and raised funds for research toward a cure, there is still much to be learned about the causes of cancer. Moreover, the true burden of environmentally induced cancer is still largely unknown.

The breast cancer movement has been quite successful at increasing disease awareness and raising funds for research and treatment. The pink ribbon has become a symbol of this success, and the American public is bombarded with images of pink ribbons, requests for donations, action alerts, and publicized declarations of women's experiences of breast cancer. The pink ribbon has become a widely recognized and popular symbol of the fight against breast cancer, and of the struggle for survival and hope. Yet, there is a darker side to the pink ribbon, as it has come to represent a form of advocacy that overlooks environmental links to cancer, and is synonymous with a consumer-based activism, which asks people to shop their way toward a cure (Klawiter 2008; Leopold 1999; Ley 2009; McCormick 2010).

Scholars such as Barbara Ehrenreich in "Welcome to Cancer Land" and Samantha King in *Pink Ribbons, Inc.* (2008) have aptly argued against the consumer-based activism of pink advocacy. This book joins the conversation about consumer-based activism and corporate involvement in health advocacy. The message adopted by pink ribbon advocacy is that we can run, walk, fund-raise, and shop our way toward a cure (Klawiter 2008; Leopold 1999; Ley 2009; McCormick 2010). This pink ribbon advocacy has been focused on research for a cure and raising awareness about lifestyle risk factors. Yet, as was pointed out by the California Breast Cancer Research Program, 50–70% of women with breast cancer have no known risk factors (CBCRP 2007). The fact that many women with breast cancer do not have risk factors indicates a need for research into the causes of cancer that can increase our knowledge about what causes cancer.

Although the pink aspect of the movement has recently begun to reframe its agenda more toward preventing cancer rather than curing it, the pink ribbons and consumer-based activism persist. I identify this aspect of the larger movement, those who use pink ribbons and adopt the strategy of consumer activism, as the "pink" part of the movement. The pink campaign's main strategy entails asking people to buy products where a portion of the proceeds goes to cancer research and the product usually features a pink ribbon. Arguably, this strategy of shopping our way out of the disease is the most controversial aspect of pink. It is controversial precisely because it often is not always clear what the money is going for or what type of research is being funded (i.e., treatment or environmental factors). Is the money being donated to an organization, which is seeking a cure, better treatment, or, for example, services for women with breast cancer? These are important questions and the details of pink ribbon products have not been transparent enough. Organizations like the Breast Cancer Fund and Breast Cancer Action (BCA) aim to be transparent and encourage other breast cancer organizations to do so, but this is an ongoing issue in the larger breast cancer movement. Moreover, corporate use of pink ribbon is not regulated in any way and therefore there is a lack of transparency regarding the way corporations are using pink ribbons, and how much money is actually being donated and for what type of research. Corporations stand to profit when they associate themselves with a charitable cause like breast cancer research (King 2004).

Therefore, corporations can benefit by placing pink ribbons on their products because it may increase their sales and therefore profits. This in itself is not necessarily problematic. However, upon closer examination of pink products it is revealed that often only a small portion of the sales is donated to breast cancer organizations and these donations tend to fund research on the pink agenda like lifestyle factors and research for a cure.

Pink ribbon products rely on a consumer philanthropy that is very profitable for corporations and there is often little transparency regarding where the money is going. Some products with pink ribbons do not identify which breast cancer organizations are receiving the money. Knowing whether any money at all is donated is crucial. For example, Oriental Trading sells pink ribbon bracelets and other trinkets like necklaces, rings, and pink pencils, yet it does not donate any money to breast cancer. In other words, Oriental Trading profits off of breast cancer without the philanthropy. Examples of pink ribbon products are everywhere, and asking questions about where the money goes and what it goes for is crucial to women's health but also the ethics of marketing women's diseases.

The lack of transparency regarding where the money goes has been an issue that the green aspect of the movement has criticized the pink for. For example, in the late 1990s, organizations such as the BCA criticized the Avon Breast Cancer 3-Day walk. BCA publicly criticized the Avon Foundation's 3-day charity walk because only 64% of the funds raised went toward breast cancer organizations, and the rest of the money was used for administrative and marketing expenses (King 2008: 53). Today Avon makes a greater effort to disclose where its money is going in an effort to increase transparency but this action only occurred after public criticism by activists such as Barbara Brenner of BCA. It has included a web link "Where the Money Goes?" for potential walkers, and it posts its financials. Through 2013 the Avon Foundation has awarded $815 million for breast cancer research (Avon Foundation 2013) and only 3% of its total expenditures in 2013 went for management and general expenses (Avon Foundation 2013). This is a significant improvement from the early days of Avon's "walk" and clearly Avon has made efforts to put more money toward breast cancer and less money toward administrative costs. The breast cancer movement has aimed to increase transparency about where the money goes and what the money is being used for. I explore the pink ribbon consumerism and transparency further in Chapter 4 where I argue how pink ribbon products are being used by the movement today and how both pink and green organizations are choosing to work with corporations.

What I term the "green" movement refers to the environmental breast cancer activism, which emerged in the 1990s. The green breast cancer advocacy is centered on challenging the use of pink ribbon products; questioning the pink movement's relentless focus on raising awareness and early detection; and demanding research into the causes of cancer, including research into the environmental links to cancer. The pink ribbon activism is also particularly concerning when you consider that companies like General Electric who manufacture mammography systems are profiting off the early detection message. Even more alarming has been pink's tendency to partner with corporations where the products are linked to causing cancer. Companies such as Yoplait and their campaign "Save Lids to Save Lives" have also come under scrutiny for using growth hormones that are linked to causing cancer. This is particularly concerning given Yoplait's alliance with breast cancer movement. Organizations like the BCA argue that this creates a circle of profit where companies contribute to disease risk while making money from health activism. This practice of pinkwashing is the norm for pink advocacy, and is embraced in the name of "finding a cure" and "raising awareness." Companies like Estée Lauder and Ford manufacture what are known as pink products, referring to a product with a pink ribbon where a portion of the proceeds goes to breast cancer organizations. In the case of Estée Lauder—which owns Clinique, Origins, La Mer, Aveda, and Bumble & Bumble, all popular cosmetic lines—many of its products have been found to contain carcinogens, formaldehyde, silica, and titanium dioxide, as well as parabens. Parabens, for example, are a group of compounds often used as a preservative and antimicrobial in creams, lotions, and other makeup products. Parabens are absorbed through the skin and is being researched for how harmful parabens are to the body and how they are linked to cancer. In fact, the Campaign for Safe Cosmetics, which is part of a coalition with Breast Cancer Fund as well as the Environmental Working Group, is deeply concerned about parabens and other chemicals in products. This book also demonstrates that pink organizations like Komen are increasingly concerned about parabens and other chemicals. Yet, it is the green organizations that go a step further, beyond demanding more research, and challenge the corrupt relationship between pink advocacy and companies whose products contain harmful chemicals linked to cancer but slap pink ribbons on their products.

Pink organizations like the Susan G. Komen Foundation and the Avon Foundation maintain corporate partnerships with General Electric, Bristol-Myers, Estée Lauder, Ford, and other corporations that directly profit off of the breast cancer industry. In fact the largest portion of Komen's budget comes from corporate partners. This is significant because the largest funders of breast cancer research include National Cancer Institute, National Institute of Health, Department of Defense, Avon, Susan G. Komen, and the American Cancer Society, to name a few (McCormick 2009). The potentially conflicting goals of corporations and advocacy organizations like Komen become an important site of the breast cancer movement to analyze. AstraZeneca's relationship to the breast cancer movement best illustrates this point. AstraZeneca manufactures tamoxifen, a cancer drug, and is also a major supporter of Komen and the National Breast Cancer Awareness Month (NBCAM). The NBCAM aims to increase awareness, and hopefully mammographies, which would lead to more breast cancer diagnoses. On the surface, this is a positive thing because it means more women might detect their breast cancer earlier; however, with more diagnoses comes more potential for profit from tamoxifen. AstraZeneca has a financial interest in cure more than prevention, as a cure is more likely to be profitable. In addition AstraZeneca is one of the top global producers of organochlorides, which are chemicals used in an array of compounds such as Agent Orange, polychlorinated biphenyls (PCBs), and dichlorodiphenyltrichloroethane (DDT). DDT for example is classified as a possible and reasonably anticipated carcinogen and an endocrine disrupter.[1] DDT has been banned in many countries.[2] Rachel Carson, author of *Silent Spring*, most aptly described the harmful impact of DDT and how it contaminates the food chain, and in turn human beings. AstraZeneca, producer of both tamoxifen and DDT, demonstrates the multiple ways it is complicit in contributing to cancer, profiting off of cancer, all the while publicly supporting breast cancer advocacy and awareness. As argued by scholars like Ehrenreich (2001), treatment is very profitable and constitutes an industry worth billions of dollars, which Brenner (2012) has referred to as the cancer industry. This book investigates how much influence corporations have over the broader cancer research agenda and over individual advocacy organizations' agendas. I find that although pink ribbons and corporate partners are highly contentious within the advocacy organizations, it is not clear that corporations directly influence the goals of advocacy organizations. Despite these findings, the politics of the pink ribbon and its form of consumer activism merits our attention as it makes visible the political economy of the disease.

In the 1990s a vibrant submovement emerged within the breast cancer movement, which questioned the pink ribbon consumer activism and demanded transparency of breast cancer organizations and what the money was being used for, while critiquing the dominant paradigm of detection and awareness. This green aspect of the movement demanded answers to questions about the environmental links to cancer. In this book I discuss the green aspect of the movement as somewhat different than the pink aspect of the movement. However, in Chapter 2, I trace these differences over time and argue that there is now a convergence between the green and pink aspects of the movement. Yet, the green aspect of the movement is highly critical about the pink ribbon and the pink campaign in general. The findings of this research demonstrate that the pink and green aspects of the movement are converging and yet pink ribbons remain a point of contention. Despite concerns about corporate influence over advocacy organizations, I find that green organizations do partner with corporations. For example, the Breast Cancer Fund, a green organization, partners with like-minded corporations such as Seventh Generation and Luna Bars. The Breast Cancer Fund has identified these particular companies as having similar principles regarding environment and toxic chemicals. In this book, I will show the ways that corporate relationships are understood by advocacy organizations and explore how they may or may not impact the agenda of an advocacy organization.

The relationship between cancer and the environment is still largely unknown and only recently has the pink aspect of the movement begun to address the role pollutants, toxic chemicals, and environmental exposures play in cancer risk and breast health. This is important because until the 1990s, when the green aspect of the movement brought this idea of cancer prevention forward, most organizations simply understood cancer risk in terms of family history and lifestyle factors. Surprisingly, only 5–10% of breast cancer diagnoses are associated with a family history of the disease, with another 15–20% of breast cancers linked to lifestyle factors, such as diet and exercise. That leaves over 70% of breast cancers largely unexplained (Massachusetts Breast Cancer Coalition [MBCC] 2015). Until recently, it was not given much credence that there were environmental links to cancer. In the 1990s, women in Long Island, New York, and Cape Cod, Massachusetts, began to notice large numbers of women with breast cancer within their communities. Activists in these particular regions demanded funding for research to investigate the role environment plays. At this moment in time, the green organizations were challenging the dominant paradigm of the breast cancer movement.

According to the MBCC, rates of breast cancer range across the state and in fact the highest rates can be found on Cape Cod (Dukes, Nantucket, and Barnstable counties), indicating a possible environmental link to cancer. In 1993, the state of Massachusetts released cancer rates by town and several advocates from the MBCC were concerned about the higher rates in Cape Cod and so they founded the Silent Spring Institute, a Massachusetts organization, which brings together physicians, public health and community advocates, and scientists to investigate chemicals and ingredients found in air, water, food, and personal care products to determine the impact toxic chemicals might have on women's breasts (Silent Spring Institute 2015). In fact in 2008, Massachusetts had the highest incidence rate of breast cancer in the United States (MBCC 2015). The existing research, such as the 2008–2009 President's Cancer Panel annual report titled "Reducing Environmental Cancer Risk," found that certain pollutants and chemicals such as PCBs, polycyclic aromatic hydrocarbons, dioxins, and organic solvents are of particular concern to human health (MBCC 2015). In fact the report states "While many Americans now carry many foreign chemicals in their bodies, women often have higher levels of many toxic and hormone-disrupting substances than do men. Some of these chemicals have been found in maternal blood, placental tissue, and breast milk samples from pregnant women who recently gave birth. Thus chemical contaminants are being passed on to the next generation, both prenatally and during breastfeeding. Some chemicals indirectly increase cancer risk by contributing to immune and endocrine dysfunction that can influence the effect of carcinogens (Reuben iii)." The fact remains that we do not know enough about the harmful effects of pollutants and chemicals on health and specifically women's risk for breast cancer. The Silent Spring Institute and other breast cancer organizations like the BCA, National Breast Cancer Coalition (NBCC), MBCC, and the Breast Cancer Fund are particularly concerned about synthetic chemicals, and the increased boom in their production and use after World War II. There are roughly 80,000 chemicals on the market in the United States and these are chemicals used in personal care and cleaning products, which most people use daily, yet the use of chemicals is largely untested (National Cancer Institute 2008–2009). The Silent Spring Institute's study "Environmental Factors in Breast

Cancer" indicated 216 compounds that were identified in causing breast tumors in animals. The study found 73 of those compounds to be present in consumer products or in food, 35 of which are air pollutants, and 25 are associated with occupational exposure (Silent Spring Institute 2007). The chemical body burden people and even newborn infants carry is of concern; in fact an average of 200 contaminants (including flame retardants and pesticides) have been found in newborn cord blood (Silent Spring Institute 2015). The Toxic Substances Control Act (TSCA) is the main law used to regulate chemicals in commerce and yet it is 38 years old and does not require companies to prove chemicals are safe before being used. TSCA is outdated but more importantly not used. There have only been five chemicals banned or regulated since 1976 under this act, and yet there are more than 85,000 chemicals on the market. The Environmental Protection Agency has only tested 200 chemicals for their health impacts. Reform of the TSCA is needed because right now the burden of proof for safety is not on companies but rather on individuals to prove that the product is harmful to their health (Breast Cancer Fund 2015). As the Silent Spring Institute's study and the President's Cancer Panel report indicate, further research and understanding is crucial to reducing cancer incidence and improving women and girls' health.

Despite the increasing number of studies that demonstrate the links between cancer and environmental exposure, most funding for cancer research is not put toward prevention. MBCC states "According to the Federal Interagency report, only about 7% of Non-Governmental Organization funding goes towards breast cancer prevention and only 10–11% of breast cancer grant funding by the National Institute of Health and Department of Defense focus on environmental health" (MBCC 2015). More funding and research are necessary if we want to truly understand the relationship between breast cancer and environment. Yet, the funding for research must shift toward a prevention-based understanding of cancer rather than focus on a cure, which has been given most attention by what I call "pink" breast cancer organizations.

The mainstream "pink" breast cancer movement has been very influential in shaping the wider research agenda toward a cure and early detection and treatment. This aspect of the movement is best represented by pink ribbons and organizations like the Susan G. Komen for the Cure and the Avon Foundation. The "green" aspect of the movement has instead focused on funding prevention-based research, and supporting legislation aimed at increasing regulation of synthetic chemicals. As a result, a clear dividing line has developed in the breast cancer advocacy world between a green environmental advocacy aimed at preventing environmental toxic exposures and preventing cancer and a pink advocacy that focuses more on fund-raising for a cure through a consumer-based activism and pink ribbons and products. Yet in the past 10 years, this dividing line has become less clear and the pink and the green are converging toward environmental prevention. In this book, I illustrate that although the movement as a whole has been moving toward increasing attention on environmental links to cancer and prevention, the politics of prevention do differ between pink and green. I trace the greening of the breast cancer movement by showing how pink organizations have come to take on environmental causes of cancer as an important part to fighting this disease.

This book extends the work of King (2004) and Kedrowski and Sarrow (2007) by arguing that although pink organizations are extremely influential, they need not be seen as dominating the movement. Although organizations like the Susan G. Komen Foundation, a national pink breast cancer organization, have tremendous public visibility and have achieved great success in fund-raising and promoting pink awareness, they have been joined by very diverse green organizations. As Sulik (2012) has argued, "Komen, however is not *the* voice of the breast cancer movement. There are other national, regional, state, and local organizations that provide the bulk of local services for diagnosed women and mobilize around diverse breast cancer issues" (50). Moving the analysis beyond pink organizations like Komen is crucial to understand the movement as a whole and the multiple ways advocates are fighting this disease. Supporting the claims of Ley (2009), I argue that green organizations have played a key role in shaping the movement's agenda toward prevention. Yet, I argue these green organizations, represented by the Breast Cancer Fund, BCA, Zero Breast Cancer, and the NBCC, no longer constitute a submovement. In fact I argue the green movement has helped shift the breast cancer discourse toward prevention and pink has followed this path. The findings of this research suggest that we are at a crucial moment in the history of breast cancer advocacy in which we see environmental breast cancer (green) and pink breast cancer organizations' interests converging toward prevention.

The scholarship of breast cancer activism in the United States begins with Montini and Ruzek's (1989) article "Overturning Orthodoxy: The Emergence of Breast Cancer Treatment Policy" and includes other major studies like Altman's *Waking Up: Fighting Back* (1996), Leopold's *A Darker Ribbon* (1999), and Potts's *Ideologies of Breast Cancer* (2000). These studies trace the history of the movement and consider the rise of breast cancer activism, its effect on policy regarding the disease, and the corresponding changes women face in terms of treatment. Although considerable literature about the breast cancer movement has extensively discussed the importance of organizations, previous scholarship has not examined either the pink or the green set of organizations as a single unit of analysis. Nor have researchers examined the ways in which the rules, principled beliefs, and internal structures of these organizations shape the strategies of the larger movement. Scholars who have examined this divide in the movement, such as Barbara Ley in *From Pink to Green* (2009), have described green breast cancer advocacy as an environmental submovement of the larger mainstream breast cancer movement, which is primarily pink. At the time of her research and book publication (Ley 2009), this approach was appropriate. However my findings show that things have changed between 2009 and 2014. Others have provided insightful in-depth analyses of the green aspect of breast cancer advocacy, including Ley (2009), Sabrina McCormick in *No Family History* (2010), and Maren Klawiter in *The Biopolitics of Breast Cancer* (2008). To those ends, this book examines three central research questions:

1. How do pink and green breast cancer organizations differ in terms of organizational policies, characteristics, internal structure, model programs, tactics, advocacies, and diversity?
2. How do these factors explain why breast cancer organizations prefer green or pink activism?
3. Are the goals of pink and green organizations converging or diverging?

Whereas much of the scholarship on breast cancer conceptually separates the pink and green movements and sees them as quite different and the green as a submovement of the mainstream pink, this study finds that they are becoming more similar and converging due to successful framing of prevention, and due to mainstream acceptance of environmental health links and the importance of prevention. Therefore, the breast cancer movement is best understood without distinguishing the pink as mainstream from the green as a submovement, precisely because the two threads of the movement are becoming increasingly similar in terms of influence and focus on environmental prevention. The data show that the differences that once existed between "pink" organizations and the "green" submovement are no longer as clear and that the "pink" is moving toward the "green." In addition to the organizational factors noted earlier, the two movements have converged for several reasons: influential scientific studies such as the President's Cancer Panel validated links between environment and cancer, pink and green are increasingly professionalized and adopt similar strategies such as citizen–science alliances, and efforts to reframe breast cancer toward environmental prevention have resonated with the general public.

As the following chapters will show, to understand the greening of the larger breast cancer movement, we must also understand the ways in which these organizations framed their activism and set their goals, and what strategies they employed. As Andrews and Edwards (2004) argued, the current literature on advocacy organizations would be enhanced by stronger qualitative research on organizations and issue domains that focuses on small and local advocacy organizations. This book aims to make such a contribution by employing a qualitative research design in place of the quantitative methods used by many advocacy and political science scholars who study social movement organizations. This qualitative research study of breast cancer advocacy organizations adds to the political science scholarship.

Research Design and Methodology

This study utilized a purely qualitative research approach to answer its research questions and assess the organizational similarities and differences between breast cancer advocacy organizations using nationally available data about breast cancer activism over the past 20 years, secondary literatures, organizational materials (Web sites, mission statements, financial documents), and 54 qualitative interviews with different stakeholders in six breast cancer organizations. In addition to the qualitative interviews, I engaged in ethnographic research from 2006 to 2013 (including participation in the annual Race for the Cure held by the Susan G. Komen Foundation from 2006 to 1012, the Avon 3-day walk for breast cancer in 2012, and several meetings held by Komen and Avon in the Boston/MetroWest area of Massachusetts and in the San Francisco area in 2012).

A qualitative research method was used to discover and understand the lived experiences of the participants and their perceptions of those experiences (Creswell 2009). Given that the purpose of the research was to present a comparative analysis between pink and green advocacy in terms of organizational attributes and characteristics, a qualitative design that could uncover those factors was the most appropriate approach for fulfilling that purpose. In-depth semi-structured interviews were particularly useful because they allowed exploration and analysis of the complexity of social movements (Blee and Taylor 2002). The interviews allow women's voices to come to the forefront and provide information-rich data about breast cancer advocacy, existing policies and programs, campaigns, decision-making processes, and organizational structures.[3]

Although there are an exceptional number of breast cancer organizations, this research focused on organizations that operated at both national and local levels, and that identified as advocacy groups. The organizations selected were purposefully chosen for the richness of qualitative data and their level of influence in the larger movement. The rationale for selecting the six breast cancer organizations was to achieve a representative sample of breast cancer organizations.[4] Furthermore, a purposeful selection of these organizations was deemed appropriate to be able to acquire in-depth information and data that will aptly address the research questions. An advocacy organization is one that "make[s] public interest claims either promoting or resisting social change that, if implemented, would conflict with the social, cultural, political, or economic interest or values of other constituencies and groups" (Andrews and Edwards 2004: 481). This is a synthesized definition that aims to link the scholarship on interest groups, social movement organizations, and nonprofit advocacy organizations. Ultimately, Andrews and Edwards (2004) argued for a synthesized definition because each of these categories is focused on "the pursuit of a collective good framed in the public interest" (485). The organizations I examine in this book are best understood in this "synthesized" way. In the field of breast cancer politics, organizations embody characteristics of interest groups, social movement organizations, and nonprofits. However, throughout this book I will refer to the organizations studied as advocacy organizations. The advocacy organizations examined in this research pursue the collective good of preventing breast cancer. After the selection of six breast cancer organizations, 30 breast cancer members/advocates were chosen through non-probability purposeful sampling (Creswell 2009). Notably, the total sample of interviewees was divided equally among the six chosen breast cancer organizations to achieve consistency in sample size, that is, five interviewees who are classified as active members/advocates from each of the six breast cancer organizations.[5]

A semi-structured focus interview guide was administered among the three main stakeholders in breast cancer organizations: (a) board of directors, (b) officers, and (c) members. Meanwhile, the primary sampling technique that was used to select the board of directors and officials for this study is nonprobability purposeful sampling. The rationale for the selection of these participants was their knowledge and experiences as stakeholders in breast cancer organizations. Although the focus of this book was on the organizations themselves, interviews of individuals who participated in and have knowledge of advocacy organizations were necessary and useful. Many of the participants in this research have been working in breast cancer advocacy for 20 plus years and have watched the movement evolve over time. They have knowledge of the larger movement and have often participated in several breast cancer organizations and therefore they could provide a unique and in-depth perspective of organizations. Feminist researchers have advocated for interviewing as a methodological technique, which (a) demonstrates a preference for unstructured and open-ended format, (b) is being open and receptive, (c) relies on careful listening, (d) is respondent-led as opposed to researcher-oriented, and (e) encourages an equal relationship between interviewee and respondent (Neuman 2006: 311). This research study has used a qualitative research design to elicit women's experiences of advocacy positions, because it sees women's perceptions and experiences as central to understanding the larger social movement of breast cancer advocacy. This study finds that viewing the breast cancer movement as embodied highlights the ways women are challenging dominant modes of thinking about disease, taking an active role in medical research and political advocacy around health care, all the while citing women's experiences of disease as a starting point for advocacy.

Embodied Health Movements

This book builds on the work of Brown et al. (2004), who argued the importance of understanding breast cancer as an "embodied health movement," stating that recent breast cancer advocacy not only demands access to health care, but also utilizes the embodied experiences of individuals as a way of pursuing its strategies. The nature of the movement as embodied is demonstrated by Chapter 2, which examines advocacy groups' focus on prevention. In Chapter 3, the movement and organizations are shown to challenge scientific findings, participating in medical research and translating medical research and scientific knowledge through the key strategy of citizen–science alliances.

Brown (2007) defined *health social movements* as "collective challenges to medical policy, public-health policy and politics, belief systems, and research and practice that include an array of formal and informal organizations, supporters, networks of cooperation, and media" (26). In accordance with the scholarship on the success of the breast cancer movement by Boemher (2000), I argue that when compared to other health-based social movements the breast cancer movement has been remarkably successful at challenging policy and shaping medical research and practice. It has also been remarkably successful at challenging people's perceptions of the disease and has brought a disease that once was silenced and held much shame and stigma into public awareness and visibility. Framing the breast cancer movement as embodied illuminates the way the breast cancer movement is moving beyond a focus on health care and access toward environment and prevention. The scope of the breast cancer movement has broadened beyond care and treatment and access to challenging the medical discourse and practice, which at times silence women and their experiential knowledge, and demanding lay people's involvement in the science, which will be examined in Chapter 3. There is an extensive review of women, the body, and breast cancer done by Laura K. Potts (2000). Potts explores "the ways in which women with breast cancer construct knowledge about their disease" (Potts 2000, 16). Potts argues that women's stories demonstrate that "biomedical knowledge" is not objective but rather informed by power relations of politics, culture, and gender. The breast cancer movement considers and values an individual's experience of illness and disease and provides an important link to the women's health movement in the United States. In an embodied health movement, participants will understand the nature of the problem through their bodily experiences and personal knowledge (Brown 2007). In the women's health movement in the United States, activists focused on the importance of valuing women's experiences of illness and their bodies as crucial to health. Green organizations like NBCC and its Massachusetts chapter MBCC are interested in taking women's bodily experiences of breast cancer as a valuable starting point for advocating for medical research. This is precisely why MBCC was involved in the creation of the Silent Spring Institute whose purpose is to research environmental links to cancer. Its research is inspired by the experiences of women living in Massachusetts and women with breast cancer who do not have a family history and are questioning environmental links to cancer. Similarly, Zero Breast Cancer was inspired by women in Marin County, California, which investigates the causes of cancer and specifically environmental factors. A senior-level advocate from Zero Breast Cancer states, "we have done community based participatory research, and we continue to be involved in this research. We actually collaborate with researchers ... we're not just summarizing research. We are actually part of the process of doing research."[6] Challenging medical research and advocating for participatory research have become cornerstones of both the pink and green aspects of the larger embodied breast cancer movement.

Ultimately, the concept of the "embodied health movement" is useful because it characterizes the way a health movement challenges the dominant paradigm of breast cancer and move toward prevention. The "dominant paradigm" of breast cancer has seen the causes of cancer as lifestyle and genetics. Today, the breast cancer movement is actively engaged in changing the dominant way of thinking toward environmental prevention.

The Way Forward

Chapter 2 examines how the framing of prevention is different within pink and green organizations as each has a different framing of prevention, coupled with a desire to build a niche within the breast cancer advocacy landscape. The central argument of Chapter 2 is that the movement toward an understanding of cancer prevention as environmental by both pink and green reflects a shift in the politics of prevention. I analyze the framing and politics of prevention in relation to organizations' desire for branding and building a niche in competitive market. Chapter 3 analyzes citizen–science alliances in both pink and green organizations, noting the importance of these alliances for the framing of prevention. Most scholarship has treated citizen–science alliances as a strategy employed only by green organizations, yet in Chapter 3, I show instead that pink and green groups alike use citizen–science alliances but for different purposes and in different ways (McCormick 2010). In Chapter 4, I examine corporate partnerships and argue this represents the biggest difference between pink and green that remains. Chapter 5 concludes the study and reflects on future directions of the breast cancer movement and research on breast cancer advocacy.

Notes

1. The endocrine disrupter hypothesis (EDH) argues that some toxic chemicals mimic the endocrine system, which can disrupt typical biomedical responses in the body and specifically breast development. Endocrine-disrupting compounds are chemicals used in everyday products like plastics, cosmetics, and cleaning products.

2. DDT was the subject of Rachel Carson's famous publication *Silent Spring*, which is considered to be a very influential book in the U.S. environmental movement.

3. In-person interviews were personally conducted that lasted from 45 to 60 minutes. However, there were interviews that were conducted over the phone, at the participant's request, that lasted from 45 to 60 minutes. I took careful notes during these phone interviews and transcribed them immediately afterward to ensure they accurately reflect the participant's views and are close to exact words. The use of coding for qualitative methods is meant to make large amounts of data more manageable by categorizing data analytically (Miles and Huberman, 1994). First, the data were coded according to descriptive concepts: history, agenda, mission, framing, tactics, internal structure, networks, and diversity as well as other themes that emerged during the interviews (Miles & Huberman, 1994). In addition, other coded concepts include (a) issue at stake, (b) location of activist events, (c) nature of event (disruptive or nondisruptive, violent or nonviolent), (d) resources, (e) target of activism, (f) environmental concerns, (g) related movement connections, (h) race and class composition, (i) prevention, (j) framing, (k) motivation, (l) objective, and (m) pinkwashing.

4. Given that the population of breast cancer advocates is large in number and diverse in terms of sociodemographic characteristics, this research delimited the selection of breast cancer advocates or members to those who are active members of pink and green breast cancer organizations within the last five years. Meanwhile, the board of directors and officials from the selected breast cancer organizations were chosen according to their position and role in the organization. These informants were selected from the same breast cancer organizations where the breast cancer activists/members will come from. This parameter was specified in order to reduce the cost of data-gathering procedures and to elucidate consistent answers pertaining to their respective organizations.

5. This research project received approval by the Institutional Review Board at the University of Massachusetts Amherst. Each participant was provided with a consent form approved by the IRB at the University of Massachusetts Amherst and asked to sign and date.

6. Anonymous, confidential interview by author, San Rafael, CA, February 10, 2011; in author's possession.

CHAPTER 2

Prevention Is a Cure

In a speech at Breast Cancer Fund (BCF) event in 2011 at San Francisco, Dr. Margaret Kripke, a member of the President's Cancer Panel, told the following anecdote:

> A physician, walking home after a long day of caring for patients, strolls along the river. He hears a voice yell out, "Help me, I'm drowning." The physician dives into the river and pulls the individual out of the water. Minutes later, he hears another voice. Again he throws himself into the water and emerges with another survivor. Soon, there is a chorus of voices calling to him from the water. Exhausted, he takes a breath before turning to jump in again. But first, he notices a basic scientist on the hill. "Come help me save these people," the physician calls to her. The physician says, "There are too many people drowning here." Thoughtfully scratching her chin, the scientist declines. "That's an interesting observation," the scientist says; "I wonder who is upstream throwing all these people in the river. I think I will head upstream to find out."[1]

Dr. Kripke's speech presented the results of the President's Cancer Panel, which found credible scientific evidence of environmental links to cancer and her story reminds us of the importance of preventing a problem rather than trying to "cure" it after the fact.

There has been a shift in the politics of prevention that entails moving away from a focus on the early detection, cure, and lifestyle risk factors toward a public health paradigm focused on environment. Organizations like Breast Cancer Action (BCA), BCF, and Zero

Breast Cancer have long focused on prevention, yet there has been a paradigm shift toward environmental prevention, which can notably be seen in pink organizations like the Susan G. Komen and Avon foundations. Building on the work of Barakso (2010) and Prakash and Gugerty (2010), these findings show that the movement toward an understanding of cancer prevention as environmental by both green and pink organizations, as traced in the previous chapter, reflects a radical shift in the politics of prevention motivated in part by branding and niche building.

The History of the Breast Cancer Movement and the Politics of Prevention

The breast cancer movement is composed of numerous breast cancer organizations around the world with a wide array of missions, resources, and information surrounding breast cancer at the global, national, and local levels. In the United States, there are many governmental agencies that are an important part of the breast cancer movement, including the National Cancer Institute (NCI), the U.S. Department of Defense (DOD), the Centers for Disease Control and Prevention (CDC), the Environmental Protection Agency, and the Food and Drug Administration (FDA), all of which play an important role in the breast cancer movement. There are also national organizations that focus on cancer more generally and also advocate for breast cancer prevention and cure, such as the American Cancer Society (ACS). In other words, the breast cancer movement is a vast conglomeration of various organizations, government agencies, and institutes. A historical overview of the breast cancer movement must view organizations as central to shaping the movement. Toward that end, my research examined organizations whose actions included fundraising, policy making, education and support, participating in institutional review boards, and conducting participant research.[2] All these advocacy organizations are highly bureaucratic, well funded, and politically connected. Organizations operating at both national and local levels have become more formalized and have increasingly adopted environmental prevention messages. Organizations with a "green" message of environmental prevention—messages that were previously more grassroots and contentious—are now more formal, and clearly professionally driven. In other words, pink organizations are becoming more similar to green, and both are now adopting a prevention-based approach. The very face of the breast cancer movement and advocacy organizations therefore has changed in an important way.

The conventional wisdom among breast cancer scholars is that the larger movement has been dominated by pink organizations and a focus on finding a cure, education, and awareness and not concerned with environmental links to cancer. Within this narrative, green breast cancer advocacy is often understood as a submovement and pink advocacy is understood as the mainstream movement (Klawiter 2008; Ley 2009). The interviews completed for this book, however, reveal a number of ways in which pink organizations have adopted a green message and appear more similar today than in the past, which indicates that the movement has changed in the past four years since the publications of Ley (2009) and Klawiter (2008). Therefore, this chapter interrogates the dominant understanding of the breast cancer movement by historically tracing the initial focus of the pink movement, the emergence of the green movement, and the increasing convergence between the two. By tracing the breast cancer movement and demonstrating its early focus on a cure as prevention, this book argues that a redefinition of prevention took shape in the late 1990s within both the pink and the green wings of the movement. The findings of this book demonstrate that rather than view the green movement as a submovement, we should acknowledge the green in the pink and the pink in the green and see both variants as part of the same movement. This new narrative, based on the results of this research, shows that pink advocacy has been shifting toward a greener understanding of prevention since 2000. The results also find that individual organizations have a central role in shaping the larger movement, and therefore, this chapter argues, organizations are crucial to the politics of prevention.

The Birth of the Pink Movement

This section traces the history of breast cancer advocacy organizations in order to assess whether at different moments in their histories, the organizations it examines adopted a green or pink message. Ultimately, it demonstrates that there has been a convergence between pink and green since 2000 and the breast cancer movement can no longer be characterized as containing a dominant mainstream pink and a secondary or submovement of green. The distinction between pink organizations as more bureaucratic and green organizations as more grassroots is no longer as accurate as it was when Ley published her research in 2009. Today, all these organizations are highly bureaucratic, well funded, and politically connected. Organizations operating on the national level and local level have become more formalized and have increasingly adopted environmental prevention messages. Organizations with a "green" message of environmental prevention that, during the second wave, were more grassroots and contentious are now more formal, professionally driven organizations. In other words, pink and green organizations are becoming more similar, and both are now adopting a prevention-based approach. The face of the breast cancer movement and advocacy organizations therefore has changed in an important way.

Breast cancer activism has a long history in the United States, dating back as early as the 1930s. This early form of breast cancer activism was largely focused on spreading awareness about breast cancer and increasing women's opportunities for early detection and treatment. In the United States, as early as the 1930s, women were organizing around the issue of breast cancer. In 1936, the Society for the Control of Cancer, which we now know as the ACS, formed the Women's Field Army (WFA) whose goal was to recruit volunteers and raise money (King 2008: xii). The WFA recruited volunteers to raise money and educate the public about cancer because cancer had primarily been a disease that was not publicly visible or discussed. The WFA focused on increasing women's education and sense of responsibility to either do self-exams or see their doctors for exams in an effort to detect cancer early. In many ways, this early activism was a grassroots movement and utilized thousands of volunteers who encouraged women to be responsible for their own health through self-exams. We see this same message articulated today by groups like the Susan G. Komen for the Cure foundation. Yet, the WFA's early organizing was very grassroots and relied solely on volunteers. It was the work of such volunteers that successfully fund-raised so that ACS could expand its reach and its membership (Anderson 2004).

Certainly, the breast cancer movement overlaps with the second wave of the women's movement and the emergence of the women's health movement in the early 1970s. The women's health movement in the United States became more widespread in the 1970s, corresponding with the growth of the women's movement and its critique of patriarchal perspectives on women's health and bodies. The women's health movement recommended that women take control of their bodies and their health. This discourse was made popular through the widely read *Our Bodies Our Selves*, published by the Boston Women's Health Collective in 1973. The women's movement encouraged women to discuss their health issues, increase their knowledge about their own bodies, and improve medical knowledge on their health issues in order to get better medical attention. These ideals were highly influential on the breast cancer movement.

It is also important to note the wider political culture of the time leading up to the second wave of the breast cancer movement. The environmental justice movement and the civil rights movement were active in the United States during this period. In 1962 Rachel Carson wrote *Silent Spring* and attributed cancer to pesticides and pollution in the environment. The Love Canal area of Niagara Falls, New York, was evacuated in 1978 after a great deal of protest from community members about high cancer rates and birth defects. It was found that toxic chemicals had been knowingly buried under the soil where their homes and schools were built. The environmental justice movement, emerging in 1982, made up predominantly of women of color, was localized and grassroots, and questioned links between environment and cancer. The environmental justice movement sparked after the state of North Carolina decided to create a hazardous waste landfill where it attempted to dump soil with toxic PCBs (polychlorinated biphenyls). Residents of Warren County were angry and concerned about the PCBs contaminating drinking water and protests ignited. Robert Bullard's (1990) work *Dumping in Dixie* was extremely influential by pointing out the locations of waste disposal facilities, most commonly found in poor communities of color. In particular, the environmental justice movement critiqued patterns of disease that were emerging in low-income communities, native communities, and communities of color. The environmental justice movement provided an analytical perspective known as environmental racism that critiqued why environmental pollution and landfills were so common in such communities (Bullard 1990). The environmental justice movement is concerned with health problems and disease incidence that are a result of environmental pollution. Therefore, breast cancer is a concern but one among many health issues linked to environment. As Steingraber noted in *Living Downstream* (1997b), an exploration of the links between cancer and the environment, this link to the environmental justice movement reminds us that breast cancer is just one of many cancers and environmental health issues. Therefore, the breast cancer movement itself is highly interconnected and influenced by other social movements of the time. The environmental justice movement and its focus on toxic pollution and its links to cancer also paved the way for breast cancer advocacy focused on environmental health.

With the vibrant women's health movement of the 1970s came a renewed focus on understanding breast cancer and reducing the public shame surrounding the disease of cancer. A policy coordinator from the BCF states,

> Sure, almost all of the organizations out there are focused on some sort of generic awareness and then raising money for either direct services or research on sort of treatment and cure; all of which is incredibly important. I think that the movement as a whole has progressed to a point where awareness is less of an issue. People are pretty much aware of breast cancer. And more and more women are feeling comfortable coming out as survivors. I think something that was sort of held as a deep secret decades ago—probably even ten years ago—has really come out into the open and has done an enormous amount to bring awareness of the issue. What we haven't made a lot of progress in the prevention side.[3]

Although breast cancer until the early 1970s was previously viewed as highly personal, advocates worked hard to frame it as a public health issue. In 1974, Betty Ford publicly announced her diagnosis in an effort to push the disease into the public eye and mainstream medical discourses (King 2004). The combination of the women's movement and its early focus on health and bodies paved the way for breast cancer's receiving more public recognition.

After, Betty Ford's announcement, the movement focused on seeing breast cancer as a social problem, not just a personal one, but it also was critical of medical practices regarding radical mastectomies. As Weisman stated, "Thus, even though breast cancer was not the leading cause of death among U.S. women, or, after 1986, even the leading *cancer* cause of death—the conditions existed in the 1980s to frame breast cancer as an important women's health problem" (2000: 218). Breast cancer was an issue that had resonance for the public despite the fact that it was not a leading cause of death. One of the concerns of breast cancer advocates was that the male medical professionals were dictating choices about treatment and mastectomy that were not in the best interest of women's health.

Breast cancer advocates fought to reduce the number of radical mastectomies using the Halsted method because other methods were proven just as effective without damaging women's bodies so severely. The treatment of breast cancer made apparent some of the glaring inequalities of health care and its attitudes toward women. One-step mastectomies, the radical Halsted mastectomy, and inadequate diagnoses were major issues for women with breast cancer during this time. As Kasper and Ferguson (2002) argued,

> As a result of the women's health movement, feminist activism, the rise of bioethics and, in the case of breast cancer, laws passed by state legislatures greater degrees of informed consent and patient autonomy gradually became components of the medical encounter. Indeed, as more women refused to consent to radical mastectomies and searched for surgeons "willing to perform more conservative and less disfiguring operations," offering procedures other than radical mastectomy had become a necessary business decision. (2002: 42)

This marks an important moment in breast cancer history because advocates were challenging medical authority and the prevailing scientific wisdom of the time (Kasper and Ferguson 2002: 41). This challenge later would become a key feature of the environmental breast cancer movement.

In 1980, poet and essayist Audre Lorde published *The Cancer Journals* (2006), which critiqued the dominant breast cancer paradigm (Ley 2009: 25). Lorde's feminist critique of the breast cancer industry and its dominant paradigms led to her refusal to wear a prosthesis after her own mastectomy. This was considered a radical position by most, due to Western culture's emphasis on the connection between a woman's breasts and her sexuality and femininity. Lorde's refusal later would inspire activists in the Bay Area to bear their mastectomy scars in public spaces and on the covers of magazines as a way of challenging the mainstream's understandings of breast cancer. The following year, Kushner's *What Every Woman Should Know about Breast Cancer* (1982) was published, critiquing the one-step process of biopsy and mastectomy. Kushner also played a key role in creating informed consent laws and would later help found the National Alliance of Breast Cancer Organizations (NABCO), a network of hundreds of organizations and advocates.

The Susan G. Komen for the Cure and the Avon Foundation are the most well-known and perhaps most influential breast cancer organizations in the United States. These organizations have a considerable amount of political influence, raise millions of dollars, and are sponsored by many successful corporations in the cosmetic and pharmaceutical industries. Their primary form of advocacy is using events like the "Race for the Cure," held in several cities across the United States and a larger event held annually in Washington, DC, to raise awareness and funds.

The Susan G. Komen for the Cure was started in 1982 by Nancy Brinker to honor the loss of her sister Susan to breast cancer. Brinker used elite political connections with key figures such as George Bush to garner support for her cause and organization. In 1983 Komen introduced physical fitness fund-raisers, what we know today as the Race for the Cure. Komen held its first race in 1983 in Dallas, Texas, and in 1990 held its first National Race for the Cure in Washington, DC. *Self* magazine and Evelyn Lauder of Estée Lauder were working on the national breast cancer awareness and wanted to use a ribbon for symbolism. After surveying women, they determined that pink is most associated with femininity and would be an ideal color for the breast cancer ribbon. In 1990 Komen gave out pink visors to cancer survivors participating in the Race for the Cure and one year later was giving out pink ribbons to every participant in New York City races, and finally in 1992 pink ribbons became the symbol of National Breast Cancer Awareness Month (Sulik 2012: 47). Pink has become a widely recognized and popular symbol of the breast cancer cause, survival, and hope.

We cannot underestimate the success of events like the Komen's Race for the Cure, which have come to be held in cities across the country, where thousands of women participate to raise millions of dollars. These events have a remarkably positive energy where the focus has always been on hope, survival, and the bonding of women. Komen's central focus in the 1990s was its emphasis on fund-raising for a cure and increasing access to mammography. The Susan G. Komen for the Cure has been very innovative in that it created a public space for breast cancer activism and raising awareness about breast cancer. The foundation has successfully brought the issue of breast cancer into the mainstream, raised millions of dollars for research, and fought for better access and funding for mammograms.[4] The success of Komen's campaign to increase awareness of breast cancer was unprecedented. Director of community initiatives at the Boston Susan G. Komen chapter reflected on the history of the movement and the success of advocates:

> The reality is that if you really look at the history of the breast cancer movement over thirty years ago, it wasn't even mentioned or publicized on TV, it wasn't part of any type of campaigning or print and newspapers. The word *breast cancer* was something that was non-existent. So if you really look at the movement of

where we have come from thirty years ago to today, you can see the difference, and that was because of the activists and advocates we had on our side ensuring it.[5]

The Susan G. Komen Foundation's success at increasing awareness of breast cancer has propelled the disease into hypervisibility.

In 1982, NABCO, best characterized as a pink organization (King 2004: xv), was formed to distribute necessary information to women living with breast cancer. NABCO serves as an early example of the relationship between breast cancer organization, corporations, and politics. As King pointed out, most of NABCO's funding came from pharmaceutical companies (xv). NABCO did not attempt to challenge the federal research agenda but rather distributed information to women and has been criticized by many scholars and advocates as showing the early problematic partnerships between corporations that profit from cancer and a movement seeking to end cancer. (NABCO disbanded in 2004, as the movement became saturated with advocacy organizations with similar focus on breast cancer awareness.) Although NABCO provides a key example of efforts to formally connect breast cancer organizations and advocates, it also fostered corporate and political relationships and did not make efforts to challenge the research agenda or to shape public policy but served more as an information-based organization where women could get up-to-date information on cancer or where women in treatment could buy such products as wigs (King 2008: xv). In particular, this key breast cancer organization did not challenge the federal research agenda as other health-based social movements such as the AIDS movement did at the time (King 2008: xv). Many of the advocates I interviewed cited the AIDS movement and its challenge to federal research as inspiring and mobilizing them and as influential in the foundation of key organizations like BCA and the National Breast Cancer Coalition (NBCC). The AIDS activist organizations used confrontational and often disruptive strategies. For example, NORCAL staged a die-in at a drug company (Kedrowski and Sarow 2007: 26). Breast cancer activists were influenced by the success the AIDS movement was having in terms of increasing funding for research and pressuring pharmaceutical companies to make particular drugs more accessible. Turshen argues that ACT UP, founded in 1987, is an example of a grassroots community response to the AIDS epidemic, which demanded that more research and treatment options be made available (Turshen 2007: 88). Klawiter (2008) stated that BCA learned a great deal from

AIDS activist organizations; she states "From ACT UP they learned how to make sense of articles in medical journals, how to work with media, how to apply pressure to pharmaceutical companies and government agencies, and how to chain themselves to the fence if all else failed" (Klawiter 2008: 173).

While breast cancer activists were witnessing the success of the AIDS movement in the late 1980s, this was also a time that the women's health movement was critical of the National Institute of Health (NIH) and its perceived tendency to fund research studies on men's diseases, using only men as participants. While Ley argues that women's health issues received less funding than men's health issues, Klawiter contends this point and argues that women's health and specifically breast cancer has always been well funded more than male cancers. Kedrowski and Sarow argue "Directing funds to breast cancer research as part of a larger women's health initiative was one way that women's health advocates would be assured that medical research funds would be directed to long-neglected women's health issues" (Kedrowski and Sarow 2007: 208).

The late 1980s and early 1990s mark an important moment for breast cancer activism in the United States, because a dividing line emerged within the breast cancer movement. This green submovement differed from the mainstream movement, which waved pink ribbons and focused primarily on fund-raising, early detection, and awareness. Ley states, "In the summer of 1990, the Congressional Caucus for Women's Issues organized hearings on the federal government's inadequate attention to women's health, including breast cancer. Second, the growth of HIV/AIDS activism prompted a dramatic increase in HIV/AIDS research during the early 1990s and sparked a move to increase funding for breast cancer research" (Ley 2009: 24). At this moment we see pink organizations like the Susan G. Komen for the Cure advocate for funding research for a cure, treatment, and early detection.

The Emergence of the Green Movement

Simultaneously with the success of the mainstream breast cancer movement, the early 1990s saw the emergence of a vibrant submovement that focused on environmental links to cancer, prevention, and challenging current medical research. It is best characterized by the emergence of several environmental breast cancer organizations such as BCF, Silent Spring Institute, West Islip Breast Cancer Coalition, and many more. This submovement fought for government-funded medical research to investigate environmental links to cancer. The 1993 Long Island Breast Cancer Study is just one example of the successes of this wing of the movement. In the face of a significantly higher-than-average incidence of breast cancer in Long Island, New York, several breast cancer groups formed in the Long Island area, including the Huntington, West Islip, Southampton Breast Cancer Coalitions and the Long Island Breast Cancer Network (Brown 2007), which have focused on the environmental risk factors of breast cancer.

A key national organization in this green submovement has been the BCA. BCA was founded in 1990 by women with breast cancer and was directly inspired by the politics of ACT UP's work on AIDS (Klawiter 2008). In October of 1990 BCA published a newsletter, which publicly criticized the ACS for its focus on a cure and treatment. In this newsletter BCA takes the stance that environmental carcinogens need to be investigated. BCA and other green organizations were frustrated with the pink ribbons and what King calls the "tyranny of cheerfulness." Klawiter argues that organizations like BCA wanted to challenge the "upbeat discourse of survival" that pink organizations had adopted (Klawiter 2008: 169). One of the ways BCA challenged this discourse was through its "Cancer Sucks" campaign. Klawiter argues that green activism was in direct conflict with pink activism at his stage. This conflict is evident in the picketing of Komen's Race for the Cure events by the Bay Area green activists. Green breast cancer activists were also in conflict with pink organizations' focus on mammograms as prevention. Barbara Brenner, former BCA president, states, "The messages the public gets about mammography are largely by the businesses and nonprofit organizations that profit from either selling products used for screening, or taking money from businesses that profit from screening. As a result, the science that has been emerging for years that says mammography should be used less is ignored or discounted by the big players" (Brenner 2012, oral history by Pluss, 15). Green organizations run campaigns like "Think before You Pink" that are meant to expose how consumer-based philanthropy campaigns do not donate sufficient amounts of money to cancer research. In addition, BCA and other organizations like the Massachusetts Breast Cancer Coalition (MBCC) have picketed the Susan G. Komen and Avon foundations for not revealing exactly where the money they have raised goes and for not allowing women from the communities in which those funds were raised to have a say in fund allocation (McCormick 2009). This critical analysis of the economics of breast cancer has been a key platform of BCA from the beginning.

A key characteristic of breast cancer organizations during the 1980s and 1990s has been an emerging focus on shaping public policy. According to Weisman,

> While the policy initiatives of the 1990s could not have happened without these organizations, it is also important to recognize that they operated in a policy content in which health care issues were salient and women's health was a popular bipartisan political issue. (2000: 214)

As Weisman describes, the 1990s held many political opportunities for developing breast cancer policy. For example, in 1990, the Breast and Cervical Cancer Mortality Prevention Act was passed. This act, initially funded with $30 million, developed mammography and pap smear test screening programs through the CDC for low-income women (Weisman 2000: 220). Early on, the Susan G. Komen for the Cure's goal was to increase access to screening methods for all women, particularly low-income women.

In 1991, the Bush administration formed the President's Commission on Breast Cancer, which was chaired by Nancy Brinker (King 2004: xv). In response to the administration's unwillingness to increase funding for breast cancer research, in 1991 Dr. Susan Love (a surgeon) and Susan Hester (a fund-raiser and activist for Lesbians with Cancer) founded the NBCC with the express purpose of influencing governmental policy regarding the disease (King 2008: xv). Early on, this coalition comprised 75 organizations including the BCA (in the San Francisco Bay Area) and the Women's Community Cancer Project (in Boston), to name just a couple. According to Weisman's (2000) account, "A planning group consisting of eight organizations soon expanded to a twenty-member working board, and by 1994, the coalition had members in all states and nearly three hundred affiliated organizations" (219). While the Susan G. Komen Foundation initially was part of the formation of the NBCC, it ultimately decided not to become a member. Klawiter articulates the impact this decision had on increasing a divide within the movement. Klawiter recounts Bay Area activists' perception of Susan G. Komen's decision "One Bay area activist told a well-known story about one of these early meetings: 'The Komen ladies, dripping in diamonds, sat on one side of the table, and across from them were some women from the Mary Helen Mautner Project for Lesbians and Cancer' " (Klawiter 2008: 139). In fact, it was speculated that the reason Susan G. Komen pulled out was because it did not wish to work with lesbians or feminists (Klawiter 2008: 139). King argued that Komen's decision not to be a member of the NBCC, which focuses on environmental causes of breast cancer and is publicly critical of the biomedical approach to breast cancer, is evidence of its conservatism as a movement (2000: 487).[6] Brenner (2002), however, argued that Susan G. Komen's decision not to become a member of NBCC was likely due to their very different agendas, as NBCC was explicitly interested in shaping policy whereas Susan G. Komen initially was not. Certainly, Susan G. Komen has forged its own path and been very successful, and more recently it has taken a more critical stance regarding prevention and established an advocacy alliance with the purpose of lobbying. Therefore, perhaps King's assessment does not hold true today as it did a decade ago. Today the NBCC has two organizational components: it is a 501(c)(4) corporation that lobbies Congress and a 501(c)(3) corporation that trains and educates advocates to work with science and health care workers. The NBCC was founded with three goals, which included promoting research on causes, treatments, and a possible cure; improving access to services; and increasing women's involvement in the issue (Weisman 2000: 219). The NBCC's growth and professionalization has resulted in a membership that in 2012 "includes hundreds of organizations and over ten thousand individuals. This coalition has been very influential and has demonstrated support for more research investigating environmental causes of breast cancer" (King 2008: xv). What is crucial to understand about the history of the movement is that although the NBCC has long held a green perspective on cancer, it is currently similar to Susan G. Komen and Avon in terms of its size, access to resources, and levels of bureaucracy. Although the NBCC continues to describe itself as a grassroots organization, its present organizational features, such as resources, size, board, and lobbyists, would indicate otherwise.

In 1991, the year of its founding, the NBCC delivered over 600,000 letters to the White House demanding more funding for breast cancer research, which occurred during the highly publicized sexual harassment accusations at the Clarence Thomas hearings (Weisman 2000: 219) that effectively put women's issues and voices in the forefront of public attention. As Weisman (2000) reported, after the contentious politics surrounding abortion and incidents such as the Anita Hill and Clarence Thomas hearings, women were elected in greater numbers in the 1992 elections. According to King (2008), in the 1992 election, many conservative politicians embraced breast cancer as an issue to wield support from women voters who were considered swing voters. As Weisman stated, "Breast cancer became the quintessential women's health issue in the 1990s that appealed to legislators regardless of their position on abortion" (2000: 217). In 1993, the Clinton administration developed an action plan in response to the Bush administration's President's Commission on Breast Cancer, and as a result screening services for low-income women were extended to all of the 50 states and mammography standards emerged. According to Weisman, "Between 1990 and 1997, federal funding for breast cancer research increased more than fivefold, from 81 million to 521 million" (2000: 222). Due to the breast cancer movement's activism, cancer research spending rose from $155 million in 1992 to $400 million in 1993 (King 2004: xvi). By 1998, the National Breast and Cervical Cancer Early Detection Program had seen an increase in funding to $145 million, $115 million more than during its debut in 1991 (Weisman 2000: 222). The Balanced Budget Act of 1997 also expanded Medicare mammography coverage. Since the mid-1980s, the primary message in the breast cancer movement has been one of early detection and searching for a cure. This focus, which was promoted by Bush's Commission on Breast Cancer, was adopted by many other advocacy organizations, as we can see best in the work of the Susan G. Komen for the Cure and in the Clinton administration's focus on screening for low-income women. At that moment in time, breast cancer as a public health issue garnered a significant amount of political support and traction. Most importantly, according to Weisman, "Breast cancer advocacy evolved from local support groups to highly professionalized national interest organizations in little more than a decade" (2002: 218).

The NBCC also includes state-level chapters like the MBCC. The MBCC was founded in 1991 by local women who were concerned about the higher rates of breast cancer in their community. High incidences of cancer in Cape Cod, Massachusetts, also led breast cancer activists there to explore the link between environmental toxins and cancer (Steingraber 1997a). According to Steingraber, "By 1993, the Massachusetts Department of Public Health had established that breast cancer in almost all the towns on Cape Cod exceeded the statewide average" (1997a: 81). Some of these women had been involved in the Cambridge Women's Community Cancer Project but wanted to focus more on policy issues (Ley 2009: 38). The MBCC initially focused on getting research funds to investigate environmental causes of cancer on Cape Cod and had success at getting Massachusetts's legislature to allocate dollars for research.

In the early 1990s, groups such as the West Islip Breast Cancer Coalition and individual activists like Lorraine Pace and Karen Miller began to map incidence of breast cancer in their Long Island community by conducting door-to-door surveys. Pace and Miller were concerned about the higher rates of breast cancer in Long Island. Breast Cancer Help, Inc., founded in 1992 by Lorraine Pace, is a Long Island–based advocacy organization that had also been involved in the mapping project.[7] The mapping projects were community-led attempts to track areas of breast cancer in Long Island, and initially suggested that neighborhoods with a cul-de-sac had higher rates of breast cancer. They focused on providing environmental education and helping to organize other mapping projects. The activism by Pace's organizations eventually led the NCI and the National Institute for Environmental Health Studies to launch the Long Island Breast Cancer Study project (Steingraber 1997a). When the Long Island study did not find any causal relationship between the chemicals tested and breast cancer, the project was criticized for being inadequate and flawed in its research design (Klawiter 2008; NCI 2010). Ley argues that some interpreted the inconclusiveness of the study to mean that environmental factors do not cause breast cancer. She cites the ACS's summary of the Long Island Breast Cancer Study project, which emphasized the questionable results due to small sample size and invalid measurements (Ley 2009: 73). The study was criticized in part for its reliance on self-reporting and an individual's ability to self report diet, medication, and lifestyle accurately and whether a layperson is aware of his or her environmental exposures (Ley 2009: 77). As a result of the inconclusiveness of the Long Island study, breast cancer activists continued doing their own research, holding scientific conferences and investigating factors that the Long Island study did not, such as drinking water (Steingraber 1997a).

Andrea Ravinett Martin, who also had breast cancer, established the BCF in 1992. In 2001, as Martin battled breast cancer, Jeanne Rizzo stepped forward to lead the BCF. Prevention, which it describes as turning science into action, became the core focus of the BCF. In fact Ley argues "Environmental breast cancer activism's growing focus on science was part of a scientific turn taken by the broader breast cancer movement—a turn that was directly influenced by the research efforts of AIDS activists in the late 1980s and early 1990s" (Ley 2009: 53). Due to BCF's focus on science, the organization's staff is made up of people with nonprofit experience, PhDs, public health professionals, and women's rights organizers. Like the Susan G. Komen for the Cure, BCF uses physical endurance events to raise funds, such as its "Climb against the Odds" and "Peak Hike." BCF also focuses on translating science for laypeople and engage in action alerts aimed at supporting policies that will protect people from unnecessary exposure to carcinogens and other toxins.

In 1993, the cover of *New York Times Magazine* featured Matuscka and her mastectomy scar was visible in a portrait titled "Beauty out of Damage." This magazine marked an important moment in the visibility of breast cancer as a public health issue. It also inspired activists in the Bay Area to bare their mastectomy scars at protests, race for the cure, and other breast cancer events. The Avon Foundation's "Crusade for the Cure" (the name was later changed to Breast Cancer Walk) was first held in 1993 (McCormick 2009). Like the Susan G. Komen, the Avon Foundation organizes events and utilizes strategies such as races, walks, and "buy pink" campaigns to raise awareness and research dollars. The Avon Foundation for Women is a 501(c)(3) public charity and has raised and donated more than $580 million worldwide for breast cancer (Introduction Meeting Avon, January 28, 2011). The Avon walk allocates funds to five specific areas: medical research, breast cancer education, early detection, clinical care, and support services.[8] It was the Avon walk that was publicly criticized by Barbara Brenner of BCA who critiqued Avon's use of money raised from the Walk for the Cure. In 1993, we see green organizations like BCA publicly criticize the pink activism of Susan G. Komen and Avon. In 1993, the BRCA1 gene mutation is discovered and, a few years later, the BRCA2 gene mutation. The discovery of the BRCA1 and BRCA2 gene mutations was very promising and became a primary focus of pink organizations for a short time. As McCormick notes there was a media frenzy over the discovery of genetic mutations that ultimately activists were disappointed by, as it became clearer that only a small percentage of cancers are due to family history (2009: 22). McCormick argues the discourse of genetics as linked to cancer is part of the mainstream biomedical approach adopted by pink organizations. Green organizations advocated research that might explain the role environmental factors play in genetic mutations. In addition, organizations like BCA have criticized that genetic testing is not widely available to women due to corporate patents by corporations like Myriad, which make it difficult for women of lower socioeconomic status to afford the test in the first place.

In 1994, with help from the MBCC, the Silent Spring Institute was founded by breast cancer survivors and advocates who began to question why they had breast cancer despite not being genetically predisposed nor considered at risk for lifestyle choices. They decided they wanted their own research institute to look at a neglected piece of the puzzle, which was environmental factors. They wanted the research to benefit their communities and women to participate in the process of research. Based out of Newton, Massachusetts, the institute offers a unique model of advocacy and science that has garnered national attention. The Silent Spring Institute has a multidisciplinary staff who work with scientists from local universities such as Harvard, Tufts, and Boston University to map cases and possible causes of breast cancer specific to the Cape Cod area and publish their research in peer-reviewed scientific journals. Its funders include NIH, National Science Foundation, Avon, MBCC, BCF, Susan G. Komen Foundation, EPA, CDC, DOD, and other public and private donors and foundations. One of a number of organizations that focuses on the environmental links to breast cancer, the Silent Spring Institute was developed in part out of the MBCC's fight for government-funded research and its goal was to have activists, survivors, and scientists working together to research environmental causes of breast cancer.

The San Francisco area has seen a similar activism based on environmental concerns. Breast cancer activism in the Bay Area began in the late 1980s and early 1990s, following a crucial report by the Northern California Cancer Center that documented significantly higher breast cancer rates in the Bay Area compared to other cities in the United States and across the globe (Klawiter 2003). Activists in this area belonging to several organizations such as BCA, Greenpeace, Women's Cancer Resource Center, and West County Toxics Coalition formed the Toxic Links Coalition in 1994, the first group in the area to link breast cancer concerns with environmental activism (Conrad and Leiter 2003). Prior to 1994, breast cancer and environmental activists had been rather isolated from each other and typically did not work together (Klawiter 2003). In 1994, we also see the Toxic Links Coalition picket the San Francisco Race for the Cure. Its decision to picket the San Francisco Race for the Cure was in direct response of Susan G. Komen's sponsorship of the National Breast Cancer Awareness Month.

Zero Breast Cancer, based in Marin County, is an important local and state-level advocacy organization in the area. It was founded in 1995 by Francine Levien and other women with breast cancer in Marin County who were worried about the high incidence rates in Marin County and San Francisco Bay Area. Initially known as Marin Breast Cancer Watch, its goal was to raise awareness and to promote scientific research on environmental links to cancer.

In 1997, Congress passed, with minimal opposition, the Stamp Out Breast Cancer Act, in which the U.S. Postal Service sold postage stamps that raised research revenue (Weisman 2000: 221). In fact, the House approved the bill by 422 to 3, and the Senate by a vote of 83 to 7 (King 2004: 70). Senator Dianne Feinstein, a Democratic senator from California, introduced the Breast Cancer Research Stamp legislation, the first U.S. postage stamp to raise funds for a special cause, which has raised $80 million since its inception in 1998 (Feinstein 2015). (Senator Feinstein has a strong record of supporting several health issues and has worked closely with several breast cancer organizations in California.) The strong support that the Stamp Out Breast Cancer Act received in both the Senate and the House demonstrates that breast cancer is not a contentious women's health issue. In fact, in 2001 the Breast Cancer Research Stamp Reauthorization Act was cosponsored by conservative Republican Senator Rick Santorum, who was also involved in sponsoring the Partial Birth Abortion Act. Santorum's support for the Breast Cancer Research Stamp Reauthorization Act demonstrates that politicians of all ideological stripes believe they can support breast cancer to improve their standing with women voters despite their position on the contentious issue of abortion. The Stamp Act was so widely supported because it was an opportunity for politicians to take credit without bearing a great deal of cost, because the funding would come from individuals purchasing the stamp. Among many lawmakers, according to King, "participation in giving, of time or money, is viewed not simply as a preferable way to fund public services, but as a vehicle for instilling civic and self-responsibility in the American people, who are understood to have become apathetic and dependent citizens" (2008: xxvii).

In 1998, Avon held a 3-day walk for breast cancer that became the subject of a great deal of criticism from organizations like BCA. Avon's event was three days and as a result it provided tents, showers, meals, and activities. BCA specifically criticized the way Avon was spending its money. For example, King notes "Participants in the first Los Angles walk, for instance, raised $7.9 million, of which only $5.02 million or 64% of the total went toward breast cancer organizations, with the remainder dedicated to administrative (including the producer's fee) and marketing expenses" (King 2004: 53). Moreover, the event required participants to raise close to $2,000 in order to participate. It was argued that only the economically privileged could even participate in this event. Barbara Brenner discusses her investigation of Avon, and her decision to submit an op-ed "Exercise Your Mind" to the *San Francisco Chronicle* led to BCA's realization that many people were concerned about where the money from Avon was going (Brenner 2012, oral history by Pluss, 22). From this critique, BCA developed its "Follow the Money" campaign. Shortly after the critical reaction to Avon's walk it decided to separate from Pallotta Teamworks that had produced the event for Avon, and announced it would create its own walk. Komen not long after hired former Pallotta employees, bought Pallotta's assets, and created a very similar three-day event (King 2004: 57). King argues that Komen's decision to buy and host a rival event demonstrates how competitive the world of breast cancer advocacy had become (King 2004: 57–58).

In 2001, Janice Barlow took over as director of Marin Breast Cancer Watch, and in 2005 it changed its name to Zero Breast Cancer. Its early work focused on the Adolescent Risk Factor Study and the Development of Breast Cancer, intended to understand if adolescent exposures and experiences might be different between women who developed breast cancer and those who did not. It collaborated with the University of California at San Francisco to pursue this study, which eventually led to further research projects. Through its Diverse Communities Outreach Program, established in 2003, it is now focusing on building coalitions with diverse groups in the Bay and Oakland areas.

An examination of organizations like BCA in the Bay Area also reveals a history of grassroots activism in their early stages. Early on, these groups were more similar to other radical organizations such as the Black Panthers, Redstockings, and ACT UP in that their goals were broad and far-reaching. In the spring of 2011 I traveled to San Francisco to conduct interviews at BCA. BCA has a small staff but their passion for their cause is unmistakable. The staff offices seem to center around a large meeting table visually signifying their commitment to egalitarian principles and decision making. BCA, despite being incredibly busy, arranged my interviews and staff members' enthusiasm and dedication to their brand were undeniable. Activists in the Bay Area whom I interviewed reported they were heavily influenced by the activism of the AIDS movement. Since then, these organizations in the Bay Area look different and their political engagement has become less about radical activist tactics and more about professionalized advocacy. In other words, the organizations themselves have become more formal and institutionalized and less grassroots. This is true as well of national-level advocacy organizations like the NBCC, Susan G. Komen for the Cure, and the Avon Foundation who all have local chapters in various cities. In addition, while some organizations were more locally focused in their early stages, several organizations such as the BCF and BCA have developed a national focus even though they remain based in the Bay Area and are very involved in local, state, and national advocacy.

As a result of this change in advocacy organizations, even the green groups examined for this book reveal a similarity in terms of function and focus to more mainstream breast cancer organizations. As a result, this book argues that these organizations no longer represent a submovement but are dominant players in the breast cancer movement. Today, they continue to investigate environmental links to breast cancer and focus on a message of prevention rather than promote early detection and a cure, yet this message of prevention is one that has been increasingly adopted by pink organizations like Avon and Susan G. Komen as well.

Since 2011, the Susan G. Komen Foundation has made a stronger effort to investigate the environmental links to cancer. Its "BPA Statement" released on October 11, 2011, is a reflection of this effort. It reads:

> Our recommendations regarding breast cancer risks are based entirely on scientific evidence and any suggestion to the contrary is simply untrue. We base our recommendations on large, well-conducted, comprehensive studies in people; the studies we rely on for any of our conclusions are fully cited on our website, komen.org ... If there is any question about a product from Komen partners or potential partner, the product is fully reviewed and carefully vetted by our Medical and Scientific Affairs team for potential links to breast cancer in people. (Komen Foundation 2011)

In many ways this is a curious statement, as it seems to reference the critiques made against Komen in 2011 that it was promoting pink products that caused cancer. Specifically it was targeted by BCA in its "Raise a Stink" campaign, which accused Komen's perfume product of containing the ingredient "fragrance," which is thought by many organizations to contain carcinogens. Komen asked the Institute of Medicine to assess current scientific findings and develop recommendations for future scientific studies. This signifies a big commitment by Susan G. Komen to engage in questions about environmental causes. The Institute of Medicine's report "Breast Cancer and the Environment: A Life Course Approach" (2011) reviewed current evidence on breast cancer and the environment and focuses on gene–environment interactions. The report makes recommendations for future research directions. This is significant because the Institute of Medicine is extremely influential in shaping the cancer research agenda and advising Congress and policy makers on health issues. As a result of the report, the Susan G. Komen Foundation's Scientific Advisory Panel has chosen three of the thirteen recommendations the Institute of Medicine has suggested for future research. Susan G. Komen has chosen to focus on studies of occupational cohorts and other highly exposed populations, new exposure assessment tools, and minimizing exposure to ionizing radiation. In other words, its funding of environmental research demonstrates its commitment to gathering scientific evidence that will support the links between cancer and environment.

In addition the Susan G. Komen Foundation has prompted its own members to take part in a dialogue about environmental links to breast cancer by distributing a survey to members. Individuals are asked to submit answers to questions such as "What are your concerns and priorities concerning environmental risk factors for breast cancer?" (Komen Foundation 2010). This demonstrates a large commitment on the part of Susan G. Komen to focus on the prevention of cancer. The Susan G. Komen for the Cure has also recently established an Advocacy Alliance, which it describes as a "nonpartisan voice for over 2.5 million breast cancer survivors and the people who love them. Our mission is to translate the Susan G. Komen for the Cure promise to end breast cancer forever into government action to discover and deliver the cures" (Komen Foundation 2009).[9]

Both Susan G. Komen and Avon foundations have increasingly been discussing, funding, and addressing environmental links to cancer. At the same time, they demonstrate more mainstream acceptance of ideas previously pursued only by the green submovement. Even more recently, the Obama administration's 2008–2009 President's Cancer Panel investigated environmental cancer risk and recommended a more pronounced focus on prevention as opposed to a cure, a focus on environmental links to cancer that is seen by many advocates at the BCF and other organizations as a "paradigm shifting" moment in time. Moreover, this book argues, this "paradigm shift" marks a moment in which pink and green organizations have become more similar and therefore their strategies and tactics have begun to overlap, as Chapter 3 will demonstrate. Moreover, the vast array of advocacy organizations in the movement has become highly organized and professional units. Today the movement is characterized not just by the pink ribbon (as promoted by organizations like Komen) but also by a particular form of advocacy that uses races, walks, and physical activity events to raise funds for breast cancer. Fund-raising has been a primary strategy of the movement in organizations like the NBCC and the Susan G. Komen alike, and has been wildly successful compared to most other health-based social movements.[10]

Framing Breast Cancer

Historically, most breast cancer advocacy organizations have framed the disease around awareness, education/early detection, and need for funding. In *The Biopolitics of Breast Cancer: Changing Cultures of Disease and Activism*, Klawiter describes the breast cancer movement in terms of cultures of action (2008: xxviii). She argued the third culture of action is one of prevention and environmental activism that is centered on reframing cancer as an environmental disease. This book extends the work of Klawiter and finds that breast cancer advocates are in the process of reframing the disease around environmental prevention and have been more successful in altering the dominant paradigm of prevention as the cure in the past 10 years. Yet pink and green advocacy organizations frame the issue of breast cancer in unique ways. Building on Goffman's (1974) understanding that framing is a means of making sense of the world, Benford and Snow (2000) referred to the process of framing as constructing meaning but distinguish three components of framing. For example, Benford and Snow argue diagnostic, prognostic, and motivational framing as separate types that represent moments where a social movement can persuade potential participants that there is a problem (diagnostic), what the best strategy is (prognostic), and why they should get involved (motivational). Framing is used by social movement organizations to articulate problems and solutions and develop strategies for activism, as well as mobilize individuals to collective action. Breast cancer advocacy organizations use frames to diagnose collective health problems, communicate views and positions, and connect to members and possible participants to each other. Breast cancer advocacy offers a successful model of frame resonance precisely because there has been a shift in understanding of prevention and a broader acceptance of green organizations' understanding of prevention in the last four years (Benford and Snow 2000; McAdam and Snow 2010; Snow et al. 1986). Benford and Snow (2000) examined how the framing of an issue can determine how well the frame resonates with people, and mobilizes individuals. They argued that successful frames draw upon shared cultural understandings (e.g., rights, morality) in order to mobilize. Similarly, in the breast cancer literature Kolker (2004) examined the ways breast cancer advocacy organizations construct meaning through framing and she builds on the work of Snow and Benford (2000). Specifically, Kolker's work is crucial for understanding the way framing helps redefine breast cancer from an individual and private problem to a collective public health issue (Klawiter 2008: 139; Kolker 2004). The results of this research project show how framing of prevention is in part motivated by a desire to carve out a niche within the competitive space of breast cancer advocacy. In this sense, this book connects the scholarship in political science on framing and the interdisciplinary scholarship on advocacy branding and niche building. The framing literature helps us explain why green is no longer a submovement as it demonstrates the success that green has had in furthering its frame of cancer prevention, as seen through pink's adoption of environmental positions and a wider acceptance of environmental links to cancer in the general public.

Finding a Cure

Historically, the mainstream pink breast cancer advocacy has fought for a cure to breast cancer, and therefore the strategy has been to increase screenings and scientific research to cure and treat cancer. However, the environmental breast cancer organizations have challenged this focus on the cure. In 2011, the communications manager at BCA questions this focus of pink advocacy on a cure. She states:

> The whole language of the cure. What does that phrase even mean? What does it mean to you? What do you think that it is? I think it is very interesting. It is about waiting, not taking responsibility, not having to take prevention. It has to be about prevention.[11]

The NBCC (a green organization) has been most successful at trying to reframe breast cancer prevention away from a focus on a cure toward an emphasis on environment. The NBCC's mission and primary goals evidence the reframing of prevention as environmental by advocates. The NBCC's mission is to:

> eradicate breast cancer by focusing on the administration, U.S. Congress, research institutions and consumer advocates on breast cancer. NBCC encourages all of those concerned about this disease to become advocates for action and change. The Coalition informs, trains, and directs patients and others in effective advocacy efforts. Nationwide, women and men are increasing awareness of breast cancer public policy by participating in legislative, scientific and regulatory decisions, promoting positive media coverage and actively working to raise public awareness. (NBCC 2012: 16)

Although its mission statement does not explicitly mention preventing or finding a cure for breast cancer, its stated "Primary Goals" are more revealing. In order to achieve its mission, the NBCC is "guided by three primary goals: research, access, and influence" (2012: 21). It desires to "promote research into the cause of, and optimal preventative and treatment interventions for breast cancer through increased federal funding, fostering innovation and collaborative approaches, and improved accountability" (NBCC 2012: 41). The NBCC advocates research into the causes of cancer in addition to treatment options. The focus on prevention is more pronounced when one examines the state-level chapter, the MBCC. MBCC's mission states, "Defining breast cancer as a political issue, the Massachusetts Breast Cancer Coalition challenges all obstacles to the eradication of the disease" (MBCC 2012: para. 19). Its stated goals are as follows:

> Create the public and political will to eradicate breast cancer, focus on environmental links to breast cancer that will lead to primary prevention of breast cancer, reject the concept of breast cancer as a chronic disease, dispel myths and misconceptions about the realities of the breast cancer epidemic, challenge the commercialization of breast cancer. (MBCC 2012: para. 10)

It goes on to state,

> We are different from other breast cancer organizations. We believe that to eradicate breast cancer we must prevent it. This does not refer to early detection in the form of self-breast exams

and mammography. We are trying to find the causes of breast cancer, so that we can prevent every woman and every man from ever getting breast cancer in the first place. (MBCC 2012: para. 3)

The NBCC and the MBCC demonstrate a commitment to prevention that is characteristic of green organizations within the breast cancer movement. Moreover, they articulate the view that they are different and that their niche is in fact prevention, which they understand as investigating the causes of breast cancer and preventing cancer before it starts. The NBCC's view of prevention is more nuanced because it includes a critique of the mainstream breast cancer movement as too pink and too complacent.

Interestingly the NBCC's (and its state chapters, like MBCC) most recent campaign the "Breast Cancer Deadline 2020" aims to "change the conversation." The goal of this campaign is to "move beyond awareness to action." It plans to focus on breast cancer prevention and preventing breast cancer metastasis. At the NBCC annual advocacy training conference's introductory meeting in 2011, the speaker asked, how do we begin to change the conversation about breast cancer? At this point a member of the audience stood up and stated, "It's too pink. Don't go to the dark side of pink and marketing strategies for the cure" (unknown participant, NBCC, 2011). The audience member was attempting to reframe the conversation about breast cancer. The NBCC purposefully wants to change the conversation from lifestyle and early detection, buying pink products, and mammograms to conversations about prevention. This sentiment was present in several of the qualitative interviews by the NBCC and MBCC members, and the view was expressed that breast cancer has been defined by corporate America and it is our time to take that definition back.

According to the NBCC the war on cancer has failed, and therefore "Changing the conversation" is more than a slogan. The NBCC feels the conversation must be changed away from a "cure" and move toward an understanding of prevention. It means that previous efforts by the movement have been unsuccessful at stopping breast cancer and therefore a change is necessary. The NBCC understands framing the conversation as a part of or step toward prevention.

A staff member at the MBCC chapter echoed this sentiment that there is a need to reclaim the way cancer is defined and understood: "Breast cancer has been defined by corporate America and it is time to take that definition back."[12] The MBCC advocate and the organization itself (MBCC and NBCC) are trying to reclaim the definition with their campaign "Changing the Conversation." The NBCC identifies this change as a need to reframe the problem, debate, and thereby change the conversation. For example, the NBCC stated, "In 1991, 119 women died of breast cancer every day. Last year, the number of daily deaths was 110. At this rate, it would take more than 500 years to end breast cancer" (NBCC Letter 2011:1). Women are more at risk today than in 1991 for example, and the stakes are high for advocacy organizations to create effective strategies if they wish to reduce the mortality rates from breast cancer in a significant way. In 2010, Fran Visco, president of the NBCC, promised that the organization would be more controversial and have new strategies and tactics. A recent campaign, the Breast Cancer Deadline 2020, is a strategy to reframe the debate of breast cancer away from individual lifestyle factors to a prevention-based model (NBCC Advocacy Training Conference Introductory Letter, 2011). The deadline aims to use tactics of political lobbying, social awareness media campaigns, and scientific training for laypeople as its primary modes for reframing the debate. The MBCC and NBCC are doing something different and challenging pink. They are not "sugar-coating" breast cancer in messages of hope and pink but are rather taking a hard stance that the environment contains pollutants that are harmful to our health. The MBCC was instrumental in the formation of the Silent Spring Institute, which would investigate the links between environment and cancer in the state of Massachusetts and specifically Cape Cod through scientific studies.[13] The MBCC's commitment to environmental prevention is evident through its support of like-minded organizations such as the Silent Spring Institute. For example, Silent Spring Institute and NBCC discuss cancer prevention in terms of eliminating toxins in drinking water, beauty products, and so on.

Susan Love's Army of Women is affiliated with the Avon Foundation. While the Avon Foundation has been slower to include an understanding of prevention in its advocacy, the Army of Women has shown a small shift toward prevention. Love stated that a large percentage of women have no risk factors and "yet we only fund research about risk factors. We don't focus on the factors that we don't know about. It has to be the culture of science that changes, the culture of industry, the culture of women, the culture of doctors. It is like we have an attitude problem."[14] This reveals to us that breast cancer advocates understand the importance of framing the nature of the problem. Love's notion that there is an attitude problem calls attention to the need for framing.

Moreover, focusing on the factors that we do not know about is a message of prevention. While she does not outright discuss environmental factors, the risk factors that we do not know about are of importance to Love and the Army of Women.

Zero Breast Cancer in Marin County has a reputation for asking tough questions about environmental links to breast cancer and helping to facilitate research into such links. Due to higher incidence rates, Zero Breast Cancer has been a very active organization in mapping projects. In 2011, at an interview, a board member spoke of the way "environment" must be expanded conceptually:

> Since we started in 1995, we have always had environment in our mission statement. So I think we were one of the earlier groups to be interested in looking at the role environment plays in breast cancer, and the initiation progression. And our definition over the years of environment has broadened out of recognition that really there are multiple causes of breast cancer and the different factors that you cannot just look at the environment without looking at genes. You cannot just look at the environment without including lifestyle and some of the traditional risk factors. So our definition is much broader than perhaps some other breast cancer advocacy groups.[15]

Zero Breast Cancer raises an interesting point that the definition of environment and therefore prevention is not static but rather constructed in different ways at different moments in time. Zero Breast Cancer's notion of prevention synthesizes the definitions offered by both pink and green organizations in that it focuses on the relationship between lifestyle, genes, and environment.

The BCF's mission states, "In response to the public health crisis of breast cancer, the Breast Cancer Fund identifies—and advocates for elimination of—the environmental and other preventable causes of the diseases" (BCF 2012: para. 3). Its vision notably includes to:

> live without fear of losing our breasts or our lives as a result of what we've eaten, touched or breathed because the environmental causes of breast cancer have been identified and eliminated; we have succeeded in informing and mobilizing a public that is unrelenting and holds government and business accountable for contaminating our bodies and our environment. (BCF 2012: 2)

BCF's mission reveals an emphasis on prevention as focused on elimi-nation of toxins in food, air, and personal care products. Specifically, BCF's mission identifies government and businesses as key players on the breast cancer prevention advocacy landscape. Prevention means stopping cancer before it starts, not curing it after someone is already sick. Several participants mentioned that it was an organization's stance on breast cancer prevention that gave them renewed passion to be an advocate to stop breast cancer and ensured their commitment to their organization. For example, a board member at the BCF described why she first got involved in advocacy but what keeps her going is the BCF's unrelenting focus on prevention.[16]

In addition, the language of prevention was seen in the organization's mission statements and public statements, and discussed as crucial by the board of directors in organizations like the BCF. An organization's focus on prevention versus the cure proved to be a significant difference between various advocacy organizations, although, there seemed to be different understandings about what the term "prevention" even means.

The goal of Massachusetts affiliate of the Susan G. Komen for the Cure is "to eradicate breast cancer by advancing research, screening, care and education. Our vision is a world without breast cancer" (Susan G. Komen for the Cure Massachusetts 2012: n.p.). It is impor-tant to note the differences between a local affiliate and the national chapter of an organization. At times, they may in fact have different foci and interpretations of their mission. Ley (2009) noted that the Massachusetts affiliate of Komen was involved in funding research on prevention while also helping to organize campaigns that challenge ads by AstraZeneca for marketing tamoxifen to healthy women. This is in contrast to Komen's national affiliate that supported the use of tamoxi-fen by healthy women. One participant from Komen, an experienced public health advocate who works at the Massachusetts chapter of Komen, emphasizes the importance of translating the impact of pro-posed legislation to its members. The Massachusetts chapter of Susan G. Komen, according to the director of community initiatives, under-stands its mission to ensure that individual constituents have an under-standing of proposed legislation and how it will affect their lives and trainings. In order to achieve this mission it uses an organizational struc-ture of funding grantees that provide trainings. This is understood as change at the local level where the grantees become the face of Komen to the community.

Early on at the Susan G. Komen for the Cure, prevention was understood in terms of lifestyle choices, early detection, and screening.

For example, the ACS informs women that being overweight, lack of exercise, having a history of taking birth control pills, and having children after the age of 30 are all lifestyle choices that may increase breast cancer risk. In this regard, prevention is understood as making smart choices about one's lifestyle and health. Risk for cancer is not just a matter of lifestyle choices, as family history and genetics do matter. Women who have a family history of breast cancer or who carry the BRCA1 and BRCA2 mutation are at higher risk. For women with this family or genetic history, prevention is often framed as the radical procedure of removing the breasts known as prophylactic mastectomy.

Klawiter (2008) identifies Susan G. Komen's focus as one of early detection, education, and screening. In this regard, early detection is understood as a form of prevention. Similarly, although some respondents reported that they chose to work with an organization like Susan G. Komen because of its emphasis on mammograms, education, and screening, a majority of respondents felt frustrated by this focus. They articulated that a focus on mammograms and screening although extremely important is simply not enough. This critique reflects the perception by some advocates that Susan G. Komen's mission is focused on the cure and individual-level factors as opposed to prevention and environmental factors. Although this may have been an accurate portrayal of Susan G. Komen in the past, very recently it has chosen to use a language of prevention and focus on environmental links to cancer. It is clear that an organization's stated principles regarding the causes of cancer affect its strategies, tactics, and outcomes.

While pink and green may have different understandings of prevention, it is clear that the idea of prevention has been framed differently at particular moments in time. The language of prevention has been used throughout the history of the breast cancer movement. Although there is evidence of changing perceptions of what constitutes cancer prevention, Wailoo (2011) makes a compelling argument that early on (1920s) cancer was understood as a threat to the white race. Wailoo argued that cancer awareness campaigns centered on the image that it was class-privileged women who were most at risk for cancer. In this sense, white upper class women had a duty to reproduce more and prevent their cancer, in the name of ensuring their race's future. Interestingly, this is an early understanding of cancer prevention that stands in stark contrast to today's understanding of prevention. In fact, Klawiter stated, "Communities of color were the primary targets of this expansion in screening programs. Mainstream discourses of breast cancer screening, in turn, were racially recoded in an effort to counteract decades of campaigning that privileged white women" (2008: 133). Screening programs were purposefully advertised in more racially diverse ways on the part of Susan G. Komen and Avon. While the advertising for Susan G. Komen and Avon uses racially diverse images in order to mobilize women to participate in walks and races for the cure, they use language that cancer affects our mothers, daughters, and wives and prevents them from being with loved ones and families. There is still a discourse of the importance of preventing cancer for the sake and future of a woman's family, thereby emphasizing reproduction. Theories about the link between breast cancer and reproduction have been hotly debated in the breast cancer advocacy community. For example, as early as the 14th century, breast cancer was called the "nun's disease" due to the perceived association with childlessness and nuns. It was perceived that nuns had breast cancer more often because they did not give birth or breast-feed. Today the association with abortion, childlessness, or delayed childbirth and with women who choose not to breast-feed still exists. McCormick argues there is still scientific dispute over all of these factors and that there is often an underlying message that women should give birth earlier and place reproduction above career and education in order to prevent breast cancer (2009: 21).

In today's environmental breast cancer advocacy community, cancer prevention is understood as stopping cancer before it starts by reducing women's exposure to environmental toxins. The early understanding of cancer prevention, Wailoo identifies, mirrors some modern-day understanding of preventing cancer through lifestyle choices that has been used primarily in the Susan G. Komen and Avon foundations. For example, Wailoo argues that in the 1930s women were expected to detect their cancer early through screening as part of their duty to reproduce. Today there is still an emphasis by pink organizations that women should prevent cancer by early detection, screening, and genetic testing so that they can be there for their husbands and daughters and fulfill their roles as mothers and wives. Therefore, there is a common narrative of understanding women's individual choices as a means of cancer prevention. This maintains that cancer is an individual disease as opposed to a collective public health problem precisely because it emphasizes the individuality of breast cancer as linked to your diet, lifestyle choices, and genes as opposed to where you live and work and your toxic exposure. Discourses of prevention are ever present in breast cancer advocacy.

Advocacy organizations such as the NBCC, BCF, and BCA articulate the view that government agencies are not doing enough to protect us from potential harm when it comes to toxins in our environment. The precautionary principle demands that government agencies such as the EPA regulate and protect us from the potential for harm. Moreover, in the face of uncertainty government agencies should act with caution. The environmental justice movement, ecofeminists, and larger environmental movements also embrace this view (Carson 1994; Steingraber 1997b). The precautionary principle has been more widely accepted in the European Union where the burden of proof is on companies to show chemicals used in products are safe for use.

Precautionary Principle

The precautionary principle seems to be a guiding force behind several organizations. The precautionary principle insists that individuals should not have to prove environmental harm but rather corporations and government agencies should have to prove there is no harm from chemicals, pollution, and other environmental factors. The green breast cancer movement has been quite influenced by this principle and has led many of its campaigns to prevent carcinogens from being placed in our personal care and food products. In fact, participants from the Zero Breast Cancer watch specifically cited the precautionary principle as important to shaping their organizational agenda. The precautionary principle as defined in the Rio Declaration on Environment and Development in 1992 reflects the principle that "Where there are threats of serious or irreversible damage, lack of scientific certainty shall not be used as a reason for postponing cost-effective measures to prevent environmental degradation" (Patel and Rushefsky 2005: 213). Patel and Rushefsky argued,

> The precautionary principle might seem like anti-science. Rather, it recognizes the limitations in the ability of the scientific enterprise to answer the kinds of questions needed for regulatory decisions. One of the important things that the precautionary principle does is to shift the burden of proof. (2005: 214)

Support for the precautionary principle is crucial to certain advocacy organizations that focus on environmental health. When asked about the role federal agencies should play, a staff member from BCA answers:

I think what is huge is that they could be doing a lot more around environment. In California, there is a Safe Chemicals Act. There is an attempt to get things to register, have the lists vetted to see if it is safe, but corporations claim trade secrets. It seems there is a lot of dancing around the scientific evidence. It's a common question we get—what is the hard scientific evidence that there is a link (between cancer and environment)? How many women need to die before we address it? Before we know something is safe, why are we dicking around with it? 35–44 million women die. We need to put patients before profits.[17]

She articulates how much uncertainty is perceived by the general public as to whether there are environmental links to cancer. A staff member at the MBCC described her own involvement in the movement as professional and personal. She had prior professional experience in health public policy but on a personal level she was diagnosed with Huntington's disease in her 20s. She saw her own disease as part of what drew her to breast cancer activism because she was more susceptible to cancer as a result of Huntington's. She spoke of the MBCC's commitment to the precautionary principle, and understands this to mean that if there is evidence of harm then it should be proven harmful before and not after the fact. As a result organizations like the MBCC support public policy that aims to hold corporations accountable to providing safe products. The precautionary principle insists that corporations need to prove their products are safe and stop hiding behind "trade secrets" as a reason not to disclose product ingredients. Similarly, a policy coordinator at the BCF states,

I'd like to see federal agencies move more aggressively in taking actions. First of all, adopt a precautionary approach. We shouldn't have to prove beyond a reasonable doubt that a chemical is dangerous before we take actions to get it out of our commerce and our world in general. So I think the sort of safety standard that we look at needs to change. And there seems to be an enormous amount of inertia. Inertia may be the wrong word. It's taking decades to evaluate chemicals and make decisions about what to do about them—decades. It's shocking to me that the study of triclosan could start in the 1970s. And we still don't have an answer.[18]

The competing definitions of cancer prevention reveal fundamental differences in various advocacy organizations' principled beliefs and missions. Ultimately, this helps us understand why advocacy organizations pursue certain strategies and tactics, which will be discussed in Chapter 3. In line with Barakso's argument, this book finds that in addition to distinct principled beliefs and missions, an organization is influenced by its internal structure and rules for decision-making strategies. However, a fuller picture of advocacy organizations must understand them as behaving like a firm in a competitive market in which they seek to carve out a niche and brand their identity. It is clear that the breast cancer movement is changing toward a greater focus on prevention and environmental factors. Therefore, the future of these advocacy organizations will depend on the way they redefine their own missions and seek to maintain their niche in the breast cancer advocacy world.

Although most breast cancer organizations claim to be guided by the science, it seems that different interpretations of that science are at the heart of the matter. Brown (2007) cites Health-Track's survey, which assessed people's views on the role environment contributes to health problems and diseases: "For breast cancer, 25 percent believed in a major role, and 39 percent in a minor role, thus giving us well more than three-quarters of those surveyed believing in an environmental role in several major health issues" (2007: 3). In other words, the movement is marked by internal debates about the causes of cancer.

Influence of Government Agencies and Panels

The President's Cancer Panel 2008–2009 has provided evidence that environmental exposures are linked to cancer and therefore some cancers are preventable, and moreover the panel importantly found that the environmental burden has been underestimated. In other words, the President's Cancer Panel acknowledges that we still do not know the true harm that environmental toxic exposures cause to our health. It concludes that government regulations are an important solution preventing cancer and reducing environmental exposure. The agenda of breast cancer organizations has most likely been influenced by previous cancer panels. For example, in 2006 the cancer panel investigated the role that healthy lifestyle choices play in causing cancer. These findings are also the perspective adopted by many breast cancer organizations such as the Susan G. Komen Foundation.

The major criticism by the breast cancer advocacy community regarding the 2006 cancer panel's report was that it did not focus on environmental factors. The release of the President's Cancer Panel report linking environmental toxins to cancer and advocating the precautionary principle was a "paradigm game changer" in the words of BCF's Jeanne Rizzo (BCF Event 2011). The guiding principle by organizations is the science and a belief in the precautionary principle.

Overwhelmingly, many breast cancer organizations focus on issues such as lifestyle. For example, examining the NCI budget reveals that less than 15% of the money goes to environmental studies of cancer. The majority of funding for cancer research focuses on the "cure" but not on the causes of cancer. It is estimated that environmental cancers account only for 6% of cancer deaths. However, Dr. Kripke, one of the three members of the cancer panel, points out that this is still a significant number of deaths and someone must speak up for these human lives (Dr. Kripke speech in February 2011 event held in San Francisco, California, sponsored by the Breast Cancer Fund) Organizations like the Collaborative on Health and Environment and BCF disseminated the panel's findings to their members and stated:

> The Panel found that the true burden of environmentally induced cancer has been grossly underestimated and that the incidence of various cancers will only continue to increase if environmental pollutants are not considered in addition to other factors that contribute to cancer, such as lifestyle choices, socioeconomic status, and genetics. (Breast Cancer Fund and the Collaborative on Health and the Environment 2010: 3)

Dr. Kripke pointed out that there is a serious inadequacy in the government's attempt to protect citizens from harmful chemicals. A staff member of the Campaign for Safe Cosmetics, which is in coalition with organizations like the BCF, argues that government agencies have been extremely ineffective.[19] She described how her mother as a scientist shaped her early interest in environmental health issues. As a result, she also works with the Alliance for Health Tomorrow, which is an environmental group based in Massachusetts. She stated,

> Right now the EPA and the FDA don't even have the power to regulate chemicals for the most part, like in the case of cosmetics.

The cosmetic industry is a fifty billion dollar industry that is virtually unregulated. There are two pieces of legislation on the books right now to regulate this huge industry and it has not been updated since 1938 [The Toxic Substance Control Act of 1976]. There are 12,500 chemicals used in cosmetics and only 10% have ever been assessed for safety. ... the FDA can't even do a mandatory recall of products right now. [20]

As she points out, the United States has adopted an inadequate response to the potential harm of chemicals in beauty and personal care products. Meanwhile, many European nations are adopting the precautionary principle. It is clear that the United States needs better regulations, as evidenced by the FDA's inability to regulate chemicals in personal care products if cancer prevention is to be taken seriously.

The findings of the President's Cancer Panel are that:

1. The impact of environmental factors is unknown.
2. There is no comprehensive strategy that exists.
3. Stronger regulation is needed.
4. Safer alternatives are needed.
5. More research is necessary.
6. Children are especially at risk.
7. Radiation exposure is increasing.
8. The military needs to address toxic exposures and the chemicals it produces.
9. If we continue to test chemicals one at a time we will never catch up.

These findings are extremely important to the "green" breast cancer advocates but have influenced the "pink" as well. It is important to note that the President's Cancer Panel received a great deal of criticism for allegedly distracting from the true causes of cancer, which are diet and smoking for example, and the second criticism is that the science is questionable regarding the link between cancer and environment because the research designs were often flawed and relied on women to self report on diet and activity. In many ways, this issue is similar to the climate change issues in that it is full of uncertainty and heated debate.

Jeanette Rizzo of the BCF identifies the cancer panel's report as "paradigm shifting."[21] Rizzo stated, "Release of the report is a historic opportunity to change the course of the war on cancer so that, in the face of the large and growing body of scientific evidence that already exists linking environmental exposures to cancer, our nation acts rather than waits for more evidence of harm. This report says, clearly, that the public needs to be protected—that we must execute a major cancer prevention strategy that protects people from what causes cancer" (Breast Cancer Fund 2011).

The Avon Foundation has provided "more than $22 million for 41 research projects focused on primary prevention, understanding the etiology and potential causes of breast cancer and developing a blood or saliva test for early detection" (Avon Foundation 2011a: 5). The Avon Foundation is interested in funding research that asks about the causes of cancer. The current slogan of the Avon Foundation is "In it to End It." According to an Avon walk promotional letter the funds raised go for screenings, support, treatment, research into causes, and prevention (Avon Foundation 2008–2011). Its other focus has been the launch of the Love/Avon Army of Women to focus on prevention by asking women to participate in research who have never had breast cancer as well as survivors. Although some participants from BCF, BCA, and Zero Breast Cancer perceived Avon's recent funding of environmental research to be suspect, they are in fact funding organizations like the Silent Spring Institute whose mission is to explicitly investigate environmental causes of cancer. Participants felt that Avon was only recently funding environmental breast cancer organizations and research because it was criticized for not caring about such causes. They expressed the view that it is inexcusable to manufacture products with chemicals linked to cancer and then endorse a pink ribbon and the fight against breast cancer. Clearly, Avon has made a decision to fund organizations like the Silent Spring Institute in order to support the diverse views of cancer prevention.

The Susan G. Komen Foundation in 2010 invested $1.25 million in the Institute of Medicine to review the scientific evidence on the role chemicals, the environment, and lifestyle play in cancer. The Komen Foundation admits that lifestyle factors have received more funding and attention than environment (Komen Foundation 2011). Yet, since 2010, it is demonstrating an increased attention toward environmental concerns. Ley (2009) argued it is important to acknowledge Susan G. Komen has had some focus on prevention and that it is crucial to see Susan G. Komen's role as multidimensional. Cancer panels and government agencies play a key role in shaping the agendas and missions of breast cancer organizations. In fact, the panel's finding that focusing on lifestyle factors without an understanding of prevention is inadequate has led to the recent shift by Susan G. Komen and Avon toward prevention. In addition, the panel's scientific credibility has validated the claims made by green breast cancer organizations and created an opportunity for pink organizations to become greener. As the science evolves, some advocacy organizations find themselves in a position where they must reframe their mission and principled statements. A board member at Zero Breast Cancer comments on Komen's recent shift:

> I don't think you could be in a breast cancer organization unless you include environment and prevention. So even the people at Susan G. Komen who've only lately jumped on the bandwagon with environment, we still don't know what their motivations are for the Institute of Medicine that they have come out with, but. ... even the American Cancer Society are just beginning to include it (environment) on their list. And I think breast cancer organizations that have just been focused on environmental chemicals are beginning to say, well, there is a genetic component. So I think in that sense there isn't a discrepancy (referring to the divide between pink and green), I think the discrepancy is actually narrowing since the movement started.[22]

When comparing these organizations it is easy to see that the Susan G. Komen for the Cure is significantly larger and better funded than other smaller national breast cancer advocacy organizations. Therefore, it has the ability to have more staff and therefore divide its work into multiple boards, councils, and teams. A Susan G. Komen staff member describes its approach:

> It is a multi-faceted approach of course we heavily depend on funds and really identify in recruiting an array of volunteers from the fundraising aspect to the grantee aspect, ensuring that those local community based organizations are supported and we as a foundation are increasing their leadership capacity so they can go ahead and develop and implement their programs but more importantly what impact they are having locally and making sure that it is a line to an array of activities. Within Komen we have different facets so you have the public relations person, you have the volunteer recruiter, you also have the person who is responsible for sponsorship and you are also cultivating those relationships

with corporate individuals. I do most of the mission work, which is the grant making education, the public policy and advocacy, and all the roles really align with one another.[23]

Throughout the interview, she emphasized how important the grantees were to fulfilling Komen's message. Komen sees grantees as strategic local-level actors who can promote its mission.

Most organizations formally have a scientific advisory council or board, as their commitment to environmental cancer prevention increases; it becomes more necessary to rely on those with scientific expertise. It is interesting to note that each of these breast cancer advocacy organizations relies on staff and board members with expertise in science, health, and activism. Parthasarathy, discussing the policy domain of breast cancer, argued that it is difficult for activists to penetrate due to the high level of expertise and scientific knowledge by actors:

The traditional participants are usually highly trained and the topics are difficult for non-experts to comprehend. Not only do stakeholders often have high levels of education and professional training, but also highly credentialed experts play particularly important roles, sitting on advisory committees that decide which drugs to approve, for example, or which chemicals are safe for public use. (2010: 356)

Parthasarathy made the compelling argument that activists are forced to obtain their own expertise over scientific knowledge and evidence and introduce their own "facts" (2010: 356). I discuss the organizational strategy of citizen–science alliances as a means of creating scientific expertise in Chapter 4. Advocates introduce their own facts by researching and investigating environmental links to cancer. This goal is reflected in their mission and this is one the primary reasons that advocacy organizations are structured around scientific advisory boards, and employ staff with PhDs and medical degrees and scientists. A senior-level policy coordinator at BCF, when asked about alliances between breast cancer organizations, responded:

I think, sadly, we have better relationships with people outside of the breast cancer movement than within because there's been not as much playing nice between breast cancer organizations. You've got sort of the big players out there. They take up a lot of space. And they're not the most progressive when it comes to looking at the new science and looking at the new stuff coming out. It takes a longer time for a bigger organization to change their strategy and movement than a smaller organization.[24]

Branding in a Competitive Advocacy Market

Barakso (2010), drawing from Gerber's (1999) book *The Populist Paradox: Interest Group Influence and the Promise of Direct Legislation*, argued that advocacy organizations are like firms in that their actions are a result of perceived costs and benefits, their niche in a larger "market" of advocacy organizations, and the desired future survival of their advocacy organization (Barakso 2010: 155). This is very much the case in the larger breast cancer movement. Organizations are striving to distinguish themselves from other advocacy organizations. Multiple interviewees discussed the desire to see their organizations as different from others, as one who truly advocates the end of cancer.

I argue in addition to understanding the way internal dynamics impact the mission and principles, it is equally important to see breast cancer advocacy organizations as seeking to distinguish themselves in a saturated market. An analysis of the qualitative interviews shows organizations have a strong desire to brand and build a niche so they may stand out among the many breast cancer organizations. Prakash and Gugerty suggested that advocacy organizations are best understood in terms of policy markets and as competing and collaborating (2010: 3), and this book extends this view. As Bloodgood stated in *Advocacy Organizations and Collective Action*,

> Advocacy organizations exist in a competitive policy market, which is likely to have a significant impact on their structures, and operations as these organizations seek to influence policy, survive, and grow. Advocacy organizations are thus guided by instrumental concerns as well as normative principles. (2010: 95)

This framework helps us to understand the emphasis on branding found in the qualitative interviews.

Prakash and Gugerty stated "We believe that while NGO actions are certainly informed by (liberal) normative concerns, NGOs also pay close attention to instrumental concerns that bear upon organizational survival and growth. They deploy resources in strategic ways and compete and cooperate with other 'firms' in the same industry" (2010: 4). The results demonstrate that in breast cancer organizations, principled beliefs regarding the precautionary principle and prevention do play an important role. However, the qualitative interviews showed it is equally important to acknowledge the ways organizations compete and cooperate with other organizations within the movement.

Barakso (2010) argued that advocacy organizations participate in a process of branding, which helps differentiate themselves among other organizations. Therefore the tactics and strategies are often a result of an organization's distinct brand. According to Barakso (2010) an organization's brand can be identified in part by its strategies and its tactics. This is evident in the case of BCA where its brand is reflected in its strategy of exposing pinkwashing and in the case of Zero Breast Cancer where its brand is using the science-advocate relationship. This process of branding does more than differentiate organizations; it provides identity and shapes strategies and tactics. The tactics of BCA for example are centered on shaming corporations or organizations who "pinkwash." "Pinkwashing" is a term coined by BCA to refer to any company or organization that uses a pink ribbon and claims to fight against breast cancer while profiting from products that are known or thought to cause cancer. BCA's brand is that it is known as the "watchdog" of the breast cancer movement and for challenging corporate profit off of breast cancer.

I argue that advocacy organizations behave like firms and are interested in their own organizational growth and survival. For example, according to one senior-level official at Zero Breast Cancer, the board actively chose a logo that did not use pink or even ribbons to distinguish the organization as a green advocacy group who works on the issue of cancer.[25] The staff and board at Zero Breast Cancer are committed to distinguishing themselves as a green cancer organization. In other words, they do not wish to be identified with the pink ribbon and the consumer-based advocacy that is associated with pink. This decision made by the board of directors at Zero Breast Cancer fundamentally shapes the way this organization is perceived by the wider public and aims to distinguish its brand from other advocacy groups' brands. The logo and their branding demonstrate the ways advocacy organizations differentiate themselves from each other. In the breast cancer advocacy world, organizations like Komen that embrace pink culture have wider recognition and acceptance. It is imperative that advocacy organizations that wish to survive in this oversaturated realm of advocacy offer a unique message that can compete with well-funded foundations like Susan G. Komen and Avon. Zero Breast Cancer does just that. Advocacy organizations must closely watch other breast cancer organizations to ensure that their brand and campaigns offer something unique. BCA is very passionate about its brand and makes sure that it is not doing similar work to other breast cancer organizations. For example, a staff member at BCA reported that "We do outreach, we go to colleges, universities, coalition partnerships, we look to see where the overlaps are in campaigns that other organizations are running or that other organizations are partnering with."[26] This helps us see that organizations are not just branding but that they view themselves in competition with other organizations and they strive to be unique with their campaigns. In order to be unique and ensure campaigns do not overlap, an organization must research like-minded organizations.

The policy coordinator at the BCF states,

> When you're sick, all you care about is getting better. There's no room for how do I clean out my house to get rid of all these products that could be bad. Or how do I prevent this disease. It's just like I wanna get better. So that's why I think the cure that Komen has branded is so powerful in a lot of ways. Because people connect with, I need to be healed. For us, it's a matter of connecting with the breast cancer community on a level of I am healed. Now how do I prevent this from reoccurring or for my daughter from getting this. I think Breast Cancer Fund has also played this sort of delicate balance between being in the environmental community but also really wanting to be entrenched in the breast cancer community.[27]

Niche Markets

Prakash and Gugerty (2010) argued that advocacy organizations are similar to firms and they function in a policy market (Bosso 2003). Breast cancer advocacy organizations also function in a policy market. In other words, breast cancer advocacy organizations must distinguish themselves and carve out a niche. The realm of breast cancer advocacy is saturated with all types of organizations. Therefore, breast cancer advocacy organizations seek to provide a unique message and therefore create a niche. Because the Susan G. Komen for the Cure and Avon Foundation are so well known and have immense resources, smaller advocacy organizations must distinguish themselves in order to survive in the market for funding and participants. In other words, smaller and less well-known organizations like Zero Breast Cancer Watch distinguish themselves as environmentally focused on cancer prevention and thus as different than larger organizations such as Susan G. Komen and Avon. As Young (2010) noted,

> If a group can quickly establish dominance, for example through strategic branding, rivals may find it difficult to challenge for members or attention from policymakers. For example, once the AARP established itself as the dominant advocacy organization for the elderly, rival organizations could only carve out niche positions on the periphery. (37)

Similarly, the Susan G. Komen Foundation has established itself as the dominant advocacy organization within the breast cancer movement. Many organizations such as BCA, BCF, and Silent Spring Institute carve out these "niche positions on the periphery" (Young 2010: 37).

Advocacy organizations attempt to create a niche in the larger market of breast cancer advocacy organizations. For example the MBCC, according to one staff member, sees itself as one of a small group of organizations that broadens the definition of what is causing cancer, whereas the larger breast cancer movement is limited to discussing lifestyles such as diet and exercise and define those as environmental risks. She states:

> MBCC is not a treatment organization. We are not a service-oriented organization. We are not funding mammography vans. We are working from a very niche level of the breast cancer moment and from our engagement with health organizations.[28]

The MBCC, as part of the larger NBCC, defines itself as a "network of hundreds of groups and tens of thousands of individuals, NBCC speaks for women ... we're not afraid to rock the boat" (NBCC 2011: para. 2). The NBCC articulates the view that advocates have an important voice in the decision-making process of cancer research and care. The NBCC fills a particular and unique role compared to other large national advocacy organizations. Specifically it wishes to include the layperson in the formation and agenda of scientific research on cancer. It feels that scientific research can benefit when women's bodies, knowledge, and experiences are considered. Its programs such as Project LEAD and its annual advocacy training conference seek to empower the individual person to play a key role in breast cancer research and policy.

Similarly, the most successful case of carving out a distinct niche in the advocacy world would be the BCA. This advocacy group serves a distinct role in the breast cancer movement as the "watchdog" of breast cancer advocacy, exposing "pinkwashing" and supporting a prevention-based message. For instance, a staff member from BCA stated:

> The brand is very in your face, we don't take any shit, we are not into pink, pink does nothing. It's a very hard, clear-cut line. We know what we stand for. Who is benefitting from the funds? What pharma companies are in bed with the organizations benefitting from the funds? Our office is small, shabby, only nine people work here. The majority of the money goes towards funding our programs.[29]

Her words clearly show the distinct brand of the BCA. The BCA distinguishes itself from other breast cancer organizations due to its strict policy on corporate donations. Its refusal to take money from anyone who profits from breast cancer is unique, even among the other organizations that are similarly focused on prevention and environmental links to cancer.

The BCF has carved out a niche for interpreting scientific findings of cancer prevention as related to personal care products and chemical toxins, while advocating state- and national-level policy solutions. It aims to translate the scientific evidence on breast cancer and environment for the public. Its mission reflects a commitment to the precautionary principle and the view that breast cancer can in fact be prevented. Its unique ability to translate science and offer practical solutions is the focus of its brand.

In the arena of breast cancer advocacy each organization plays a distinct role. Breast cancer advocacy organizations exist within a larger arena of the breast cancer movement and actors such as government agencies and panels. Often advocacy organizations seek to carve out niches in order to differentiate themselves. According to Barakso,

> In this view, interest groups may foster their brand and contrast their group with others in their larger issue sector (say, environmental policy) by establishing their expertise in a narrow subset

of issues that they seek to be identified with (such as saving a particular endangered species). (2010: 161)

This has been the case with the BCA where it focuses on the more specific issue of pinkwashing and prevention. Ultimately the BCA sees these issues as linked. It supports the California Safe Chemicals Act and wants to "put patients before profits," according to, a staff person at the BCA. Similarly, the BCF has shown its expertise in interpreting cutting-edge science on the links between cancer and the environment. Therefore, in order to ensure success and pursuit of principled goals, advocacy organizations must brand themselves while also being aware of government agencies' and panels' actions and statements in order to revise their mission at times and guide their five-year strategic plans.

Whereas the Susan G. Komen and Avon foundations have distinguished themselves as primarily fund-raising organizations whose goal is to contribute to cancer research, they are also distinguishable by their pink ribbon branding and their focus on the "cure." In fact, Susan G. Komen recently changed its official name to Susan G. Komen for the Cure. This helped solidify the unique role that Komen plays in the breast cancer advocacy world. However, it is important to view Susan G. Komen, Avon, and other breast cancer organizations as competing for resources in a market. As King has stated,

> Thus, in a situation that is somewhat analogous to the effect of stores such as Wal-Mart and Target on small business owners, organizations such as Avon and the Komen Foundation are competing for donor-participants with smaller, community-based organizations, a situation that is particularly problematic in cities like San Francisco, which in 2003 played host to a Race for the Cure, A Breast Cancer 3 Day, and an Avon Walk for Breast Cancer, all in the space of three months. (2008: 59)

In this sense, advocacy groups often behave like firms in competition for limited resources in a saturated market. A former chair of the board of directors at the BCF describes why she initially got involved at BCF and how prevention came onto the agenda:

> I was working with the founder, Andrea. She was an inspiration to me. Andrea was a young woman and diagnosed twice and I was very inspired by her. She was key to other people. She was

very passionate. In 1997, the organization (BCF) functioned as a support group and raised awareness. It was a lot less focused than we are now. It struck me, about Andrea, that she was concerned and angry. She was asking the question why did I get this disease? Why, I am a young woman, and this is wrong. This is a very different perspective than the American Cancer Society or the Komen Foundation. Andrea was focused on the why. In 2001, the board of directors re-focused its mission and Andrea was part of the reformed strategic plan to not focus on research. She cared about this and no other organization was doing this. In 2001, we took stock of the competitive landscape and we saw that some organizations were focused on mammography, others research, and others support. At the time it was a risk to focus on prevention but it has really blossomed in the past few years.[30]

Her comments are quite revealing. BCF began by asking questions about why some women get cancer and desired to focus on prevention. BCF chose to "take stock of the competitive landscape," which means that it understood the importance of branding, distinguishing itself from other organizations, and saw itself as competing with firms, as Barakso's work suggests.

Advocacy organizations are emphasizing environmental links to cancer and using citizen–science alliances to prevent cancer. Each advocacy organization seeks to build a niche and as a result defines prevention in particular ways. A close examination of advocacy organizations shows that pink organizations are shifting toward prevention that accounts for lifestyle, early detection, and environment. In other words, the pink is becoming more and more green, thereby representing a significant change in the movement as a whole.

Notes

1. Notes for speech by Dr. Margaret Kripke, San Francisco, CA, February 2011, in author's possession.

2. Although many service and care-based breast cancer organizations that provide support groups, wig fittings, meal drop-offs, and financial aid to women fighting breast cancer are also an important part of the breast cancer movement and crucial to women living with breast cancer, those organizations fall outside the focus of this study.

3. Anonymous and confidential interview by author, San Francisco, CA, February 10, 2011; in author's possession.

4. The "Race for the Cure" in the District of Columbia was estimated to raise $3.5 million in 2010 (Komen 2010). According to McCormick (2009), all the events raised over $96 million in 2004 (49). For example, Komen's 3-Day for the Cure has raised $500 million since 2003, which funds research and community programs that focus on education, screening, and treatment (Susan G. Komen Foundation 2011). For the 3-day event, participants must raise a minimum of $2,300 and pay a registration of $90. The foundation holds events in 14 cities, including Boston and San Francisco. In 2010, the Boston event raised $4 million on Facebook alone (Meeting Notes Introduction in Milford for Komen 3-Day). The foundation has made a great effort to provide mammograms to low-income women. In other words, Avon and Komen have had significant success at fund-raising by hosting events like races and walks.

5. Anonymous, confidential interview by author, Boston, MA, November 17, 2010; in author's possession.

6. The NBCC seems to be positioned in the middle of the political spectrum, to the left of organizations like Komen and to the right of groups like BCA. In addition, many of Komen's corporate sponsors like Chevron and Estée Lauder are the very companies critiqued by environmental breast cancer activists. Interestingly green breast cancer activist groups like BCA out of San Francisco refuse donations from corporations that make money off of breast cancer like General Electric (GE), which manufactures mammogram machines. Komen foundation is sponsored by GE and many pharmaceutical companies that produce tamoxifen (a breast cancer treatment drug) (Swissler 2003).

7. Today Breast Cancer Help, INC. is also a member of the NBCC.

8. The Silent Spring Institute, which is devoted to breast cancer prevention research, received $200,000 from the Avon Foundation to further research environmental causes linked to breast cancer (Avon Foundation 2011b). Avon Boston's largest donation is to Massachusetts General Hospital, which received $750,000 for research and communicating and distributing information about care services (Avon Foundation 2011b). Avon San Francisco walk raised $5.5 million in 2009 and the funds went to University of California San Francisco Comprehensive Cancer Center and the San Francisco General Hospital partnership $20.2 million in 2010. Other funding goes to the NIEHS/NCI "Breast Cancer and the Environment Research Centers" ($1.16 million) and Zero Breast Cancer ($1,092,500 since 2003), which investigates environmental causes of breast cancer. Even though Avon funds environmental research, the overwhelming amount of Avon's dollars goes to research stages of breast cancer and markers of risk, as well as medical care for underserved populations (Avon Foundation Support in Northern California through 2010).

9. Chief executive officer and founder Nancy G. Brinker runs Susan G. Komen for the Cure. The Komen Foundation leadership also consists of

a chair of the board, board of directors (nine members), leadership team (twelve members), scientific advisory board (six members), six advisory councils (eight members each), and Susan G. Komen for the Cure ambassadors (one), and the affiliate network (consisting of 126 offices located all over the United States and the world).

10. Breast cancer receives more funding than any other cancer. According to the NCI, by 2005 the funding level for breast cancer was $560.1 million and prostate cancer was $309 million. Funding for ovarian cancer was $97.7 million in 2005. Compared to other women's diseases and other cancers in general, breast cancer received substantially more support. This demonstrates that not only is breast cancer winning out over other women's health issues such as heart disease and reproductive rights but it is also at the top of the list compared to other cancers. Breast cancer is currently receiving an enormous amount of funds for research, the majority of which comes from federal funds. The NIH, the CDC, and the DOD collectively spend $850 million on breast cancer research.

11. Anonymous, confidential interview by author, San Francisco, CA, February 8, 2011; in author's possession.

12. Anonymous, confidential interview by author, Boston, MA, November 16, 2010; in author's possession.

13. The Avon Breast Cancer Crusade states its desire for "supporting cutting-edge research to find a cure for or prevent breast cancer as well as programs that enable all patients to access quality care. Funding supports awareness and education: screening and diagnosis; access to treatment; support services; and scientific research" (Avon Foundation 2011b, para. 4). The support for prevention has since translated into Avon's active commitment to fund organizations like the Silent Spring Institute, which promote the precautionary principle.

14. Notes of Dr. Susan Love's speech, NBCC Advocacy Training, Washington, DC, May 2011; in author's possession.

15. Anonymous, confidential interview by author, San Rafael, CA, February 10, 2011; in author's possession.

16. Anonymous, confidential interview by author, phone, March 20, 2011; in author's possession.

17. Anonymous, confidential interview by author, San Francisco, CA, February 8, 2011; in author's possession.

18. Triclosan is an antibacterial chemical and endocrine disruptor that is typically found in soap, toothpaste, and cosmetics.

19. Anonymous, confidential interview by author, Jamaica Plain, MA, November 5, 2010; in author's possession.

20. Anonymous, confidential interview by author, Jamaica Plain, MA, November 5, 2010; in author's possession.

21. Notes for speech by Jeanette Rizzo of Breast Cancer Fund, Dr. Kripke event, San Francisco, CA, February 2011; in author's possession.

22. Anonymous, confidential interview by author, San Rafael, CA, February 10, 2011; in author's possession.

23. Anonymous, confidential interview by author, Boston, MA, November 17, 2010; in author's possession.

24. Anonymous, confidential interview by author, San Francisco, CA, February 10, 2011; in author's possession.

25. Anonymous, confidential interview by author, San Rafael, CA, February 10, 2011; in author's possession.

26. Anonymous, confidential interview by author, San Francisco, CA, February 8, 2011; in author's possession.

27. Anonymous, interview by author, San Francisco, CA, February 10, 2011; in author's possession.

28. Anonymous, confidential interview by author, Boston, MA, November 16, 2010; in author's possession.

29. Anonymous, confidential interview by author, San Francisco, CA, February 8, 2011; in author's possession.

30. Anonymous, confidential interview by author, phone, March 20, 2011; in author's possession.

CHAPTER 3

Citizen–Science Alliances

At a National Breast Cancer Coalition (NBCC) advocacy training conference, Joy Simha, cofounder of the Young Survival Coalition (YSC), observed,

> The status quo isn't good enough. We honor women by admitting that we don't have answers to all of the questions but we will not be successful until we do. We have to continue to help and monitor health care reform. What I see happening now is that scientists and advocates are working together to formulate strategies together and advocates need to be at the table.[1]

The YSC is an organization specifically for young women who are diagnosed with cancer. Although YSC was not an organization focused on in this book, it is a key organization in the movement and is a strong presence at the NBCC's advocacy training conference. The NBCC's annual advocacy training conference brings together laypeople, scientists, and advocacy leaders in the movement in order to learn effective advocacy strategies and get up-to-date information on cutting-edge cancer research and public policy that might impact the fight against cancer. The conference itself is an example of the types of relationships being built between citizen advocates and scientists. Simha's comments highlight a key strategy used by breast cancer advocates, one that sees the relationships between scientists and advocates as key to the success of the movement. This chapter presents a key research finding: that breast cancer advocacy organizations use citizen–science alliances to pursue their understanding of prevention. A close examination of breast cancer advocacy organizations' strategies and tactics reveals a focus on building citizen–science alliances, translating and disseminating scientific research on breast cancer, and utilizing online tools and organizational coalitions and networking to pursue their overarching belief in prevention. The focus on prevention discussed in Chapter 2 has directly influenced the strategies and tactics adopted by advocacy organizations, and in this chapter, I argue that the strategies of advocacy organizations and their tendency toward tactics that use scientific knowledge-building expertise and disseminating scientific information together represent evidence of the convergence between pink and green. At the same time, the results of this study also show that pink and green organizations use citizen–science alliances in somewhat different ways, as best shown in the example of Bisphenol A (BPA) campaigns. I also show how Web-based activity such as Webinars, action alerts, and blogs are key tactics used to disseminate scientific information. Moreover, I examine calls for participatory research designs as part of the effort to use citizen–science alliances to shape policy and change toward environmental prevention.

Creating Scientific Knowledge and Expertise

In *Mobilizing Science*, McCormick argues that some social movements seek to democratize science where the goal is to change the "methods, content, institutions, or political impacts of science" (2009: 33). The primary strategy for achieving these goals is to ensure that laypeople and activists should have a seat at the table and become active participants in the realm of scientific research. The supporting strategies include encouraging women's participation in medical research, translating relevant scientific findings for laypeople, funding, and engaging in prevention research. The findings of this research show that organizations are heavily influenced by scientific research and are looking for ways to translate information as well as take part in shaping the cancer research agenda.

Citizen–Science Alliances

Citizen–science alliances refer to the relationships and collaborations between laypeople (citizens) and scientists. A layperson is someone without professional or specialized knowledge and instead relies on his or her embodied experiences of disease as a starting point for building knowledge. According to Brown, the laypeople involved in citizen–science alliances are typically members of a toxic-waste group or environmental group, yet the findings of this book tell a different story than Brown posits (Brown 2007: xv). The findings of this book indicate that citizen–science alliances are a key strategy used by both pink and green aspects of the breast cancer movement, and not necessarily members of a clearly defined environmental group or green breast cancer group. In other words, evidence of pink organizations using this particular strategy of citizen–science alliances suggests that these alliances are not necessarily made up of only an environmental group, but rather members of an impacted health group.

Regardless, citizen–science alliances represent a key effective strategy used by breast cancer advocates from both pink and green aspects of the movement. Brown described the key advocacy strategy of "citizen–science alliances" as incredibly powerful (2007: xiv):

> Their work has led to new scientific data, major shifts in scientific thinking, valuable challenges to science policy, and a vibrant environmental health movement that has consolidated the best characteristics of the civil rights, women's, environmental, environmental justice, and other movements. (2007: xv)

The true impact of these alliances and the specific mechanisms of their effectiveness remain to be measured. In *Mobilizing Science*, McCormick (2009) has completed a study, investigating and comparing the environmental breast cancer movement to the anti-dam movement in Brazil as a means of assessing citizen–science alliances' true impact. Brown (2007) argues that citizen–science alliances are powerful and influence the mainstream paradigms of disease. The findings of this research also contribute to this conversation in that they demonstrate that advocates believe citizen–science alliances to be an effective strategy for influencing science policy and creating new ways of thinking about breast cancer. For example, one participant who is active in several breast cancer groups and has completed the NBCC's Lead Training and is a Susan G. Komen advocate in science states,

> So as advocates we want to see all the disciplines working together because we're seeing everybody in their silos doing their own track of research without enough interconnections as to where we're going. And so stand up for cancer, which you know is a Hollywood based thing, or it was. It's now associated with the American Cancer Research Institute, tried to get these dream teams together so that the research would be working together. But because of the nature of academia, from what I can see, is that every researcher or scientist is judged on how many papers

they produce. And so you know they just are becoming a paper churning out mill, maybe their papers aren't actually helping as far as breast cancer. One hopes they are but sometimes you worry that there's just this kind of network to keep churning out more of the same. And so the Department of Defense (DOD) tends to want to work more on idea, awards, thinking outside the box type of thing because there's a frustration in the breast cancer community that we've had this war on cancer since Nixon's day or whatever and we haven't got anywhere, or not very far.[2]

Advocates have the opportunity, as this participant argued, to encourage researchers and the Department of Defense to fund innovative research. The participants' comments also demonstrate the growing frustration among advocates that the war on cancer is not being won.

Ultimately breast cancer advocates use the strategy of "citizen–science alliances" because they perceive that scientific research has not been serving the needs and agendas of those actually affected by breast cancer. As the participant discussed, "there's a frustration in the breast cancer community that we've had this war on cancer since Nixon's day or whatever and we haven't got anywhere, or not very far."[3] In other words, advocates demand that scientific research serve the needs of the vulnerable and impacted. Mary K. Anglin (1997), in "Working from the Inside Out," discusses the prevalence of women with breast cancer who articulate the view that women with breast cancer should be involved in the medical research's agenda setting. Scholars like Anglin and advocates alike feel that women with breast cancer should be playing a role in shaping the cancer research agenda. Organizations like the NBCC state that "The focus on research has involved working consistently year after year to ensure adequate Federal appropriations for high-quality, peer-reviewed research. But in addition, National Breast Cancer Coalition has been committed to making sure those hard-won research funds are well-spent, and that relevant research in the private sector addresses the needs of breast cancer patients" (NBCC 2015). Citizens can shape the research agenda in many ways, including asking scientists to consider the impact their research has on women with breast cancer, asking new questions to encourage scientific innovation, and challenging and/or supporting policy related to breast cancer. The findings of this research indicate that advocacy organizations are using citizen–science alliances to translate science, train laypeople in scientific approaches to disease, and encourage participatory research.

Translating Science

McCormick identifies citizen–science alliances' method of knowledge-sharing as "Discussion and deconstruction of official knowledge; countering of expert and lay claims" (2009: 7). Citizen–science alliances aim to take on "official knowledge" or scientific expert knowledge and make it accessible for laypeople while simultaneously challenging or countering some scientific claims. Translating the science is a primary goal of breast cancer advocacy groups like the Breast Cancer Fund (BCF), Zero Breast Cancer, and NBCC, all of which desire to make scientific knowledge and expertise available to laypeople. For example, the BCF's Web site states, "We translate the growing body of scientific evidence linking breast cancer and environmental exposures into public education and advocacy campaigns that protect our health and reduce breast cancer risk" (BCF 2015). Similarly, the NBCC sees one of its key roles as interpreting and translating the latest scientific evidence. For example, the NBCC states,

> NBCC's website provides easy access for the public to up-to-date information on breast cancer issues and news of the day, with the more in-depth, patient-centered perspective ... NBCC's website is also the place to find analyses and fact sheets on recent developments in research and public policy that provide an informed, educated, and unbiased advocate perspective to emerging breast cancer issues. (NBCC 2015)

The NBCC and the BCF demonstrate the ways advocacy organizations engage with scientific knowledge. Staying on top of current research findings and challenging some of the sensationalized media coverage of breast cancer from a scientific view are important roles to be played by organizations like the NBCC, particularly for women with breast cancer who are searching for answers about how to fight their disease.

Contestable Disease

When asked whether there were disputes about the causes of breast cancer, one participant stated,

> Well I know there is a debate and I think some of it is manufactured because the idea that we can only find that there is certain cause and effect and cause and effect is such a black and white thing that we can point to ... breast cancer is just this really

complicated orchestra of different factors, so to say there is a cause and effect is just simply not true. Obviously some people carry genes that pre-expose them to breast cancer. I would never argue otherwise, but there has been way too much focus on genetic and lifestyle choices which are also usually presented in a way that blames the victim so are you obese, do you not exercise, do you smoke, have you had an abortion, um and those are also issues that we need to talk about but I think that the way that the tone and they frame it is pretty disturbing.[4]

This participant hints at the tendency to frame cancer risk in a tone that seems to blame victims or in other words blame the women who get cancer as having done something wrong. This participant is disturbed by this patter and wants to draw our attention to the complexity of cancer risk.

Cancer is a complex disease as this participant discusses, and to think of the causes as an "orchestra of different factors" is a useful way to think through both the disease and the competing discourses about cancer risk. The participant calls attention to the fact that while cancer is complex with an array of different factors, some risk factors get more attention from the breast cancer movement. A focus on genetic predisposition and lifestyle has dominated the pink aspect of the movement for some time, as discussed in Chapter 2. Yet, this participant also suggests that some of the framing about cancer risk is in danger of becoming a rhetoric of victim blaming, where what women do or do not do is to be blamed for their cancer. This type of thinking does more than blame those with cancer as somehow causing cancer, but also shifts the discourse away from a public health understanding of the disease and rather individualizes this disease.

The public health perspective of breast cancer demands an examination of structural conditions and environmental factors that contribute to health inequality. Former chair of the board of directors at BCF in 2011 reacted to the scientific controversy around cancer and environment:

A lot of people dispute the causes of cancer. We are a lone wolf in that we argue the environment is linked to cancer. People often say prove it but you can't because it is not a simple cause and effect. We know that it is in our products and we can extrapolate a link. There is controversy in the scientific method of proving harm. We believe in the precautionary principle. There are some who focused on genetic predisposition but the consensus is that it is a small percentage.[5]

Her comments remind us of the complexities of proving a link between cancer and the environment. Because of these complexities, it would seem understandable that an advocacy organizational strategy would revolve around interpreting and translating science to its membership base and potential members, and as seen in her comments, BCF is interested in opening up the conversation beyond genetic predisposition.

One participant from a green organization states,

> Well, I think different organizations I think came to the realization of the complexity of causes for breast cancer at different periods of time. But I see most really informed organizations are broadening into the environment and we've been here fifteen years and there was really a time that saying the environment playing a role, well that was really very crazy and nuts to some. But now I don't think you could be a researcher and I don't think you could be in a breast cancer organization unless you include all of that, and so even people like Susan G. Komen who've only lately jumped on the band wagon with the environment because we still don't know what their motivations are for the IOM, what they've come out with, but ... and even the American Cancer Society are just beginning to have a ... are beginning to include in their list. And I think breast cancer organizations that have just been focused on environmental chemicals are also beginning to say, well, there is a genetic component. There is ... so I think in that sense there isn't a discrepancy. I think the discrepancy actually narrowing since the movement started.[6]

The idea that the paradigm has shifted away from a narrow understanding as cancer caused by genetic predisposition and lifestyle factors toward environment and a nuanced view that environment might impact genetic makeup is a clear demonstration of the shifting conversation, but also evidence that pink organizations like Susan G. Komen are moving toward a focus on environmental prevention.

Brown argued that "Controversies over scientific research in breast cancer take place in three arenas that constitute the process of fact making and knowledge production: doing scientific research, interpreting science, and acting on science" (2007: 48). Scientific research on breast cancer and environment can be understood as such an arena of contestation because the causal links between environment and cancer are often not directly clear, and as the former board member from the BCF has stated, it is not a simple cause-and-effect relationship.

Interpreting science, as Brown argues, is a key step in advocacy aimed at prevention. Citizen–science alliances have been key to advocating for research into environmental links to cancer and also discussing the complexity of proving a causal relationship between environment and cancer in part because it is difficult to measure exposure over time. Julia Brody, executive director of the Silent Spring Institute, discussed this difficulty at the NBCC advocacy conference.[7] Brody states there is no gold standard for measuring exposure. First you can rely on self-reporting and ask individuals questions about where they work, age of onset of menstruation, and so on, yet Brody argues that looking at where a person lives is a more helpful question to get at issues of air and water pollution. Environmental measures would be examining the dust and air in the home, for example. This is an area where Silent Spring Institute is very interested. Brody also discusses the challenge of human studies where you might use biomarkers like hair, fingernails, blood, and urine but these types of studies are costly and difficult because they span across the lifecycle. Brody is making the point that breast cancer causation is complex with multiple factors that cross the life span and this can make it more difficult to create research designs that ask the right questions. This is best demonstrated by the inconclusive findings of the Long Island Breast Cancer Study. In fact Brody states that Long Island may have left people with the impression that the study found nothing but this is simply not true. The Long Island study did give results but they were not as definitive as many had hoped. Critics of Long Island study may question the proof of links between environment and cancer, yet as Chapter 2 notes, the precautionary principle and the President's Cancer Panel suggest that we need not wait for proof but rather strength of evidence, and we do have that now. Interpreting science is a key role that advocacy organizations through citizen–science alliances can play.

Interpreting Science: The Long Island Study

The importance of interpreting and translating science for changing the breast cancer agenda is best seen through a close examination of the Long Island Breast Cancer Study. In the 1990s the environmental breast cancer movement, what I call green, emerged in part due to growing concerns about higher cancer incidence in some communities of the United States where the laypeople were observing cancer clusters. Communities primarily in Long Island, New York, the Bay area of California, and the Cape Cod area of Massachusetts demanded the government research the connections between environmental toxins and cancer (Brody et al. 2005: 2). Brody et al. discuss the way these three regions played an active role in the design of the research studies and in increasing transparency of medical research, as well as setting the agenda for scientific research of breast cancer including getting a "legislative mandate" to investigate environmental links to breast cancer (Brody et al. 2005: 4–10). In breast cancer advocacy there is a push to see women's knowledge of their bodies, environment, health, and science as equally important to scientific and medical knowledge. We best see this in the case of Long Island where women first noticed alarming incidence of breast cancer and suspected environmental causes. This ultimately led to government-funded research (Long Island Breast Cancer Study) to determine the relationship between environment and cancer in Long Island.

Women in Long Island began mobilizing first in order to understand the nature of their problem and get an accurate sense of how many women had breast cancer and also where they lived. Women living in Long Island began to form groups and a plan to map the cases of breast cancer, in order to identify a pattern (Brown 2007: 77). Several advocacy groups in the area were formed such as the Huntington, West Islip, and Southampton Breast cancer coalitions and the Long Island Breast Cancer Network (Brown 2007: 77). It is this very activism that persuaded the National Cancer Institute (NCI) and the National Institute of Environmental Health Studies (NIEHS) to launch the Long Island Breast Cancer Study Project (LIBCSP; Steingraber 1997a: 80). This case demonstrates the impact health-based social movements have, as well as the need for a breast cancer movement that places emphasis on environmental risk factors.

The LIBCSP, beginning in 1993, investigated possible environmental causes of breast cancer in Suffolk, Nassau, and Schoharie counties of New York and Tolland County, Connecticut. The LIBCSP was funded by the NCI along with the NIEHS. The study examined body burden levels of compounds such as DDT (dichlorodiphenyltrichloroethane), DDE (1,1-Dichloro-2, 2-BIS (p-Chlorophenyl) ethylene) PCBs (polychlorinated biphenyls), chlordane, and dieldrin. The findings of this

study were not able to conclusively determine that exposure to organo-
chlorine compounds was associated with the elevated risk for breast
cancer. The findings were not able to rule out the possibility that
breast cancer risk is elevated from exposure. Although the findings could
not conclusively state that environmental factors are related to risk of
cancer, the results of the study did open up new areas for future studies
(NCI 2008).

Interpreting Science: Cape Cod, Massachusetts

High incidences of cancer in the Cape Cod also spawned breast cancer
activists interested in exploring the link between environmental toxins
and cancer (Steingraber 1997a: 81). Steingraber (1997a) states,
"By 1993, the Massachusetts Department of Public Health had established that breast cancer in almost all the towns on Cape Cod exceeded
the statewide average" (Steingraber 1997a: 81). Advocates demanded
further studies, which ultimately led to the Upper Cape Study and the
Cape Cod Breast Cancer and the Environment Study (Steingraber
1997a: 81). In Massachusetts, advocacy organizations like the
Massachusetts Breast Cancer Coalition (MBCC), a state chapter of the
NBCC, and the Silent Spring Institute have focused on funding and
designing research studies that investigate environmental links to cancer.

Interpreting Science: San Francisco, California

The San Francisco Bay Area of California has seen a similar activism
as Cape Cod, Massachusetts, and Long Island, New York. As early
as the 1990s, advocacy in California has been very influenced by the
AIDS activism movement and environmental justice movement.[8]
Organizations like the BCF, Zero Breast Cancer, and Breast Cancer
Action (BCA) are all based out of California and have had tremendous
influence in the greening of the breast cancer movement. In addition to
demanding more research into environmental links to cancer, organizations like BCA and BCF have drawn attention to corporate influence
on the larger breast cancer movement.

Translating Science: The Case of Bisphenol A

Despite the contestation over breast cancer causes, BCF aims to
increase knowledge and publish scientific information in ways that
laypeople can understand the relationship between cancer and disease.
The organizational emphasis on translating science is most evident in

BCF's publication, *State of the Evidence: The Connection between Breast Cancer and the Environment*, 6th edition. This publication provides an in-depth summary of up-to-date scientific evidence linking chemical exposures in our environment with breast cancer risk. The BCF offers online versions of the publication in an effort to make the science as accessible as possible. The policy coordinator at BCF states,

> We publish a biannual report called State of the Evidence. And that really sets for us what we should be working on. Because you look at the evidence of what's out there in consumer products in the environment that's linked to breast cancer. And that's what we focus on. I think that's been the tool that the Breast Cancer Fund has used to decide where we're gonna go and what we're gonna do. So that's what brought us into Bisphenol A and what's brought us into some work on phthalates.

Although the former chair of the board at BCF articulates the view that breast cancer is not a simple cause-and-effect relationship, there are other reasons for disputes about cancer. Brown (2007) argues it would necessitate corporations changing their behavior. Brown provides insight into why environmental links to health are disputed:

> Environmental health is so strongly contested because the hazards identified by laypeople and some scientists are crucial parts of the modern economy, and the challengers seek to level the playing field by having corporations be more responsible. In addition, environmental health activism poses a philosophical challenge by arguing for a people-centered society rather than one dominated by profit seeking without regard for consequences. (2007: 2)

Breast cancer advocacy often identifies hazards that ask corporations to be more responsible, which could affect corporate profits. Take for example the BCF's recent campaign to eliminate BPA in baby products and canned food. BPA is one of the most common household chemicals, and has been declared a reproductive hazard by some states. BPA is a very common chemical that we are exposed to everyday. For example, BPA can be found in food and drink containers, thermal receipts, eyeglasses, and some plastics. BPA is an unstable compound and leach seeking; it can leach into products (especially when these products are heated). For example, food cans are lined with an epoxy resin that has BPA. The lining helps to prevent bacterial contamination in food products, yet the BPA can also leach from the epoxy resin into the food. The BCF has had some success in having corporations like General Mills change their production to eliminate BPA, yet there must also be intervention from federal agencies. BPA levels can be found in our bodies (blood, urine, and breast milk) as a result of using products with BPA. BPA has also been found in placental tissue and umbilical cord blood (Environmental Working Group 2009; Schonfelder et al. 2002). It is a health concern for multiple reasons as it increases risk for breast cancer, prostate cancer, infertility, early puberty, metabolic disorders, miscarriage, and type-2 diabetes (BCF 2014). A policy coordinator at the BCF discusses the need for federal agencies to play an active role. She uses BPA as an example of such an opportunity. She states:

> One of the big issues that we work on here is Bisphenol A—this chemical that's in hard plastics but also in our food. And the biggest hurdle to having the federal government do something to prevent this is that the FDA doesn't have the authority to change the current regulatory system with which they regulate food packaging.[9]

The BCF built "citizen–science" alliances to demonstrate and translate the credible evidence that BPA in products contains carcinogens. Its concrete strategies revolved around targeting corporations like Campbell's and General Mills to remove BPA from canned food goods. Ultimately, the BCF strategy was twofold because it also focused on state policy–level solutions that would remove BPA from products, while creating action alerts to petition corporations like Campbell's to change their behavior. The campaign against BPA has been extremely successful. The mainstream acceptance today that BPA is linked to cancer and the current marketing of baby and infant products as BPA-free demonstrates the success of the BCF's strategy. Former chair of the board of directors at BCF discussed the success of the BPA campaign and the role that state and federal agencies have to play:

> There are two big things that we have been working on recently. BPA and endocrine disrupters in the environment. We have worked very hard for many years to legislate. We have had a lot of luck at state levels and many states have banned BPA. We tried to introduce it as a federal bill with Feinstein. We are

also working on the canned food campaign, which is a huge market and we have had a lot of push back. We have had people on a diet without BPA and found that their levels dropped. We can see the effect that market changes have had. A few years ago water bottles and baby bottles had BPA. The market responded faster to our concerns than the legislation, so we worked on both.[10]

The ban on BPA from baby products has become accepted by the general public, as evidence by most of the products found in baby stores and articles in parenting magazines acknowledging the importance of BPA-free products for infants and children. Ultimately, the ban on BPA in baby bottles did require citizen–science alliances in order to translate the scientific knowledge to the general public. Because this is such a contested debate it is highly important that advocacy organizations build these citizen–science alliances in order to advance their mission of prevention and change policy toward cancer prevention. Initially, BPA was not thought to be very dangerous, yet efforts by advocacy groups were able to demonstrate the harmful effects of BPA. At the time of the interview, this participant was the deputy director for Safer Chemicals, which is part of a coalition with BCF and BCA, among hundreds of other organizations. Reflecting on the larger impact BPA has on the movement, she stated:

I work on BPA linked to breast cancer and prostate cancer. This is one chemical that we use to tell a broader story of chemicals in order to garner public support and lobby Congress. For example, BPA works in grassroots. Activists use BPA as a story piece to lobby Congress and the CDC to show 93% of Americans show BPA in their bodies. This is an opportunity to prevent cancer and ask Congress to reform out of date laws.[11]

The BPA campaign represents a successful advocacy strategy aimed at shifting the debate toward prevention. Eleven states in the United States have restricted BPA in baby products. In June 2013, Senator Dianne Feinstein (D-CA) introduced the BPA in Food Packaging Right to Know Act. This act requires labeling of all food that contains BPA. Similarly, 13 states in the United States have proposed legislation that either bans or requires labeling of BPA in food products. Like the United States, Belgium and Denmark have banned BPA from infant products. Yet, we have still not seen a ban on BPA in adult products like food packaging.

In 2010 Susan G. Komen posted a statement saying BPA has been deemed safe (Komen Foundation 2010). In 2011, Susan G. Komen denied the link between environmental pollutants, toxic chemicals, and cancer risk (Komen Foundation 2011). Since 2011, the Komen Foundation has made a stronger effort to investigate the environmental links to cancer. Its "BPA Statement" released on October 11, 2011, is a reflection of this effort, which reads:

> Our recommendations regarding breast cancer risks are based entirely on scientific evidence and any suggestion to the contrary is simply untrue. We base our recommendations on large, well-conducted, comprehensive studies in people; the studies we rely on for any of our conclusions are fully cited on our website, komen.org. … If there is any question about a product from Komen partners or potential partner, the product is fully reviewed and carefully vetted by our Medical and Scientific Affairs team for potential links to breast cancer in people. (Komen 2011)

In many ways this is a curious statement, as it seems to reference the critiques made against Komen in 2011 that it was promoting pink products that caused cancer, such as its Promise Me perfume. This perfume was widely criticized for containing toxic chemicals linked to cancer. The Promise Me perfume was the centerpiece of an action alert by the BCA where 5,000 people sent letters to Susan G. Komen urging it to recall the perfume and sign a pledge regarding its use of toxic chemicals in products. Ultimately in 2011, Susan G. Komen agreed to reformulate the perfume. The context and timing of the action alert alongside the conversations about BPA represent a pattern of reluctance in Susan G. Komen's willingness to tackle toxic chemicals as linked to cancer. Susan G. Komen's statements about BPA and environmental links to cancer even contradict the President's Cancer Panel report released in 2010. Yet, Susan G. Komen in 2013 offered the environmental challenge grants in order to better understand environmental factors. This was largely in response to the Institute of Medicine's 2012 report "Breast Cancer and the Environment: A Life Course Approach." Komen is using its grant program to fund research into environmental causes of cancer. For example, Komen announced that California research organizations will receive $4.5 million to understand environmental factors. The policy coordinator at BCF reflects on the recent shift by Susan G. Komen and states,

Komen for the Cure has sponsored a panel by the Institute of Medicine on breast cancer and the environment. So they have done whatever one does to sponsor and create this committee. So clearly, it's an issue that they're hearing about—they want to know more about it, and something's clearly pushing them to sort of take that position—and the same with the National Breast Cancer Coalition. They did a bill that created more research. I think the difference between those efforts and initiative and ours is that we looked at the science. We've studied the science. We've compiled the science. And we strongly believe that there is more than enough there to take action.

Advocacy organizations often take on the role of disseminating complex scientific information. Braun argues that there exists a complex relationship between laypeople, advocacy organizations, and scientific experts. She stated: "In these models, the goal is to transfer information or advice from scientists to the public, with the media often employed to popularize expert knowledge" (2003: 193). The use of citizen–science alliances is significant. Komen chooses a top-down approach and as such struggles with what scientific information to disseminate, and will only post scientific findings that have been corroborated by federal agencies and studies like the President's Cancer Panel. Organizations like the BCF are committed to the role laypeople have in shaping the research agenda and determining activist strategies, and they are committed to disseminating scientific knowledge. The case of BPA represents this type of relationship.

Translating Science: Social Networking and Web-Based Strategies

Breast cancer advocacy organizations are interpreting and translating scientific findings and one of their primary tactics is to convey the information through the use of online action alerts, Webinars, blogs, and Facebook, which offer a cost-effective way to fulfill an organization's mission. After an advocacy organization determines interpretations of the latest scientific studies, it is tasked with finding ways to translate this to laypeople and disseminate crucial findings to its potential audience. One such way to do this is with traditional print materials that may also be offered online. The BCF has produced documents such as "The State of the Evidence" with this very goal in mind. In addition, the policy coordinator at the BCF states, "We do a lot of organizing online, Facebook, and tweeting, and email actions" (BCF 2010).

In addition to print publications, most breast cancer advocacy organizations engage in some type of online-based strategies such as Webinars, Listservs, blogs, online action alerts, petitions, and newsletters. For example, the BCA communications manager emphasizes the organization's use of online tactics such as petitions, Facebook, social networking, twitter, blogs, blog conferences, press releases, and Webinars. These tools are used to reach a wide audience and disseminate an organization's mission and current campaign. This strategy of online approaches is quite common in the breast cancer movement.

The Susan G. Komen for the Cure also uses Web-based tools to disseminate the most recent medical research, extensive information about the disease of breast cancer, and the latest treatment options. In fact, it uses its Web site primarily for education and outreach. In a sense, this is strikingly similar to the more green organizations, which use their Web sites for education and updates on the latest scientific findings.

Avon's primary strategy has been to raise funds for research and therefore shape the larger breast cancer research agenda. Therefore, its online strategies are mostly geared toward individual-level fund-raising as opposed to Webinars, action alerts, and petitions. For example, a participant in an Avon event such as "In It to End It Walk" receives a personalized Web site, e-mail reminders, templates for fund-raising, e-mail signature links to fund-raising, and Facebook fund-raising tools. Avon sees online tools as crucial to successful fund-raising and therefore participation in the breast cancer movement. This in turn shapes a primary tactic of organizations like Avon and Susan G. Komen, which is to use consumer-based strategies, corporate donors, and fund-raising events to raise funds for breast cancer research.

Zero Breast Cancer organization uses e-mail lists to disseminate some of the latest scientific findings. A staff member states,

The more we try to disseminate, translate and disseminate the research but it's primarily through an email list. We have an email list of about five thousand. So people are actually interested in the research from our organization. So when there's a study published we'll do a press release. We'll summarize the study. We'll link it to—so just providing the information I guess to various groups, a wide range of groups. . . . So we're trying to reach people in a variety of ways. We've started using social media. We just did a review of the literature in social media, and how to use it for several reasons. One to retention in young girls who are adolescent research studies for collecting real time data and then for dissemination and translation, so how can you disseminate research, translate and disseminate to wide audiences? So that's kind of been a focus.[12]

E-mail lists, Web sites, social media, and Webinars remain a key way to translate and disseminate scientific information. The goal is to reach as wide an audience as possible and to make the science accessible to laypeople.

Scientific Training

Training laypeople into advocates and active participants in scientific research decision making is a key component of citizen–science alliances and the promise of prevention. The NBCC has used a specific and unique model to prepare advocates to participate in scientific research decision making. Its Project LEAD has been quite successful in this regard. Project LEAD (Leadership, Education, and Advocacy Development) is a program where laypeople can participate in workshops on breast cancer led by experts. This prepares laypeople to sit on review panels, grant-making boards, and other locations where decisions about breast cancer are made. According to Joy Simha, one of the cofounders of YSC and presenter at the NBCC advocacy training conference, "scientists and advocates are working together to formulate strategies together and advocates need to be at the table. We can do that because we have taken project LEAD" (NBCC 2011–2012).

The Susan G. Komen for the Cure also trains advocates in science, so that it may review grants and advocates can shape the research agenda. Many advocates participate in several breast cancer organizations and therefore membership and action cross the boundaries of organizations, as advocates obtain different resources and information from whatever the niche of that organization is. The Bay Area Cancer Connections: Breast & Ovarian Cancer Information & Support (formerly called Breast Cancer Connections) located in Palo Alto, California, is primarily focused on services and support and has a vision of being a community-based cancer center who partners with the medical community and collaborative organizations while addressing gaps in cancer services. At Breast Cancer Connections, several volunteers, staff, and board members saw their advocacy spanning across several of the organizations featured in this study. For example, while working at Breast Cancer Connections, one advocate discussed how she had completed the training to be a Komen advocate in science and the NBCC trainings like Project LEAD.[13] In other words, she felt the training offered by Komen and NBCC were invaluable and that both were truly necessary. She states "The National Breast Cancer Coalition, I was drawn to them because of their training modules that they have a week long in depth science training and that is initially what brought me to them. Komen you know, it is very splintered, like I'm interested in the science also besides the patient advocacy end of things so I joined Komen Advocates in Science because they review grants for the Department of Defense which has all of the money for breast cancer."[14]

Participatory Research

Advocates desire not only to have a seat at the table and shape the focus of breast cancer research, but also to advocate women to increase their participation in medical research trials. Dr. Susan Love, founder of the Avon/Army of Women and speaker at the NBCC advocacy training conference, commented on the success of NBCC and the need for women to participate in research:

It was one thing to wear pink and raise money and that is all good but if we want to stop breast cancer then we have to have a plan. The NBCC has always been at the forefront of this. If we launch and push forward and demand and yell and scream and join the Army of Women then we can. We can't tell them we want more research and then have no women who will be a part of it. (NBCC 2011–2012)

In addition, groups like the Dr. Susan Love Foundation (and the Army of Women) and Zero Breast Cancer aim to influence the scientific research being done on breast cancer. The Army of Women is a program of the Dr. Susan Love Research Foundation that was founded in partnership with the Avon Foundation for Women. The Army of Women aims to partner women and men with researchers so that more research can be done into the causes of breast cancer. Dr. Susan Love, a key leader in the breast cancer movement in addition to creating her own foundation, has also worked with the NBCC. In Love's view,

Science has moved us forward but this doesn't always translate. Mammography is not prevention even though we know that we haven't changed the clinical arena. There are still people who are stuck in the early detection message only and we've got to figure out how to translate and bring along the medical profession, which is incredibly conservative.[15]

Love demonstrates a flaw in pink organizations' understanding of prevention as mammography and early detection. Love suggests that we move beyond this message of early detection and awareness and follow the science toward environmental prevention. As discussed in Chapter 2, organizations like the NBCC, BCA, Zero Breast Cancer, and BCF maintain there is credible evidence of environmental links to cancer. Therefore they advocate policy and research that acknowledge the links between cancer and environment. As outlined in Chapter 2, until recently, organizations like Susan G. Komen and even Avon have shown an unwillingness to understand cancer prevention as environmentally caused. While there are still disputes over the environmental links to cancer many studies such as the President's Cancer Panel 2008–2009 have found ample evidence of the role toxic exposures play in causing cancer. Yet even among advocate members of pink and green organizations the disputes of cancer were acknowledged as concerning.

The strategy employed by the Army of Women is to ask women to participate in the medical research trials that aim to understand cancer and breast cancer treatment more fully. However it is not clear whether the Army of Women is an example of citizen–science alliances because the Army of Women sees women as passive participants in the medical research process as opposed to active agents who shape the agenda. In other words, in the larger environmental movement, women are encouraged to become participants in research studies, have a seat on the decision-making bodies regarding research, and receive scientific training to translate the latest scientific medical research studies for their memberships. Yet in Love's formulation of advocacy, women are asked to participate in studies but keep power dynamics intact where scientists and doctors shape the larger cancer research agenda. According to Ley,

At one end of the spectrum, activists participate—often in small but significant ways—in studies already designed and approved by research officials. At the other end, activists are involved in "community-based participatory research," an innovative approach that emphasizes "active and equal" collaboration between lay citizens and scientific investigators from the very beginning of a study's design to the dissemination of its results and development of interventions. (2009: 57)

We must then examine the ways that advocacy organizations choose to disseminate scientific findings. Zero Breast Cancer does more than disseminate scientific information; it, like Susan Love, feels it is important to engage in community-based participatory research. According to a staff member at Zero Breast Cancer,

We're one of the only organizations who really have done community based participatory research. And we continue to be involved in this research. So we actually collaborate with researchers who are doing the research. We don't just summarize research. We are actually part of the process of doing research.[16]

A close look at the strategy of the NBCC reveals a focus on the scientific education of advocates and laypersons. The NBCC aims to be involved in decision making in hospital boardrooms and scientific grant making. A staff member from Zero Breast Cancer organization states,

We're one of only organizations really who—of the breast cancer organizations that I can think of who really have done community based participatory research. And we continue to be involved in this research. So we actually collaborate with researchers, we're not just summarizing research. We actually are part of the process of doing the research.

Community-based participatory research is a key form that citizen–science alliances take and is of crucial importance to shape the breast cancer research paradigm toward prevention. The long history of green and pink groups advocating for community-based research is a significant attribute of breast cancer activism.

Participatory Research: Fracking and Breast Cancer

Fracking has quite recently become of central importance to breast cancer advocates and has in the past five years entered onto the agenda of breast cancer organizations like BCF and BCA. Organizations like

BCF and BCA are concerned about the growing body of evidence linking fracking to numerous environmental health issues but specifically increasing risk of breast cancer. Hydraulic fracturing or fracking is an industrial method of accessing natural gas that involves heavy use and transport of water and chemicals. Fracking has often been cited as a potential solution to our pressing environmental sustainability and energy concerns by offering the United States a bountiful domestic energy source that will reduce dependence on foreign oil, stimulate the U.S. economy, and form the centerpiece of a new national energy plan. It has been criticized by environmentalists principally for its mistreatment of land and as an example of corporate greed and exploitation at the expense of the environment. Fracking takes place in many states in the United States such as Oklahoma, Pennsylvania, and North Dakota to name a few, while other states have banned or passed a moratorium on fracking in response to the growing concern about the safety of fracking.

A 2011 study commissioned by the U.S. House of Representatives found that many of the 700 chemicals used in fracking were "chemicals of concern," including benzene, acrylamide, ethylene oxide, BPA, and formaldehyde (Environmental Protection Agency 2012a; 2012b; 2014a). The threats these chemicals pose include water contamination, air pollution, and occupational hazards because "underground injection is the most common method of disposing fluids or other substances from shale gas extraction operations," leading the Environmental Protection Agency to examine various disposal methods and their safety (Environmental Protection Agency 2014a). Fracking has entered onto the agenda of breast cancer groups and demonstrates the links between environmental harm and degradation, health, and cancer risk.

Common symptoms reported among those who live near fracking sites include fatigue, burning eyes, dermatologic irritation, and headaches; upper respiratory, GI, musculoskeletal, neurologic, immunologic, sensory, vascular, bone marrow, endocrine, and urologic problems; endocrine disruption; and changes in the quality of life and sense of well-being (McDermott-Levy et al. 2013: 45). Fracking has also been linked to cancer and other health issues such as nervous, immune, and cardiovascular system problems (BCA 2014a). Despite a level of scientific uncertainty, however, there is enough evidence to suggest that fracking is correlated with particular health problems in communities where fracking occurs (Environmental Protection Agency 2014a). In 2011, the Centers for Disease Control and Prevention reported six counties in the western Dallas-Fort Worth area as having the highest rates of breast cancer in Texas. These same counties are the ones involved in fracking. Similarly the Texas Cancer Registry reports an increase of cancer in these counties. The BCA is concerned about higher incidences of breast cancer in Texas's six counties where there is intensive gas drilling (BCA 2014b).[17] According to the U.S. Committee on Energy and Commerce, companies have used products (fracking fluid) containing known carcinogens. The committee reports "Between 2005 and 2009, the oil and gas service companies used hydraulic fracturing products containing 29 chemicals that are known or possible human carcinogens, regulated under the Safe Drinking Water Act (SDWA) for their risks to human health, or listed as hazardous air pollutants under the Clean Air Act" (Committee on Energy and Commerce, Democrats 2011). The same report finds that benzene, toluene, xylene, and ethylbenzene are found in the fracking injection fluid. Benzene in particular has been classified by the Environmental Protection Agency as a Group A human carcinogen. The Institute of Medicine's 2011 report links breast cancer to benzene, 1,3-butadiene, and ethylene oxide, all of which can be found in gasoline fumes, vehicle exhaust, tobacco smoke, and some occupational settings (Institute of Medicine 2011).

In addition many chemicals in fracking fluids are known endocrine-disrupters and exposure has also been linked to breast cancer. The Environmental Protection Agency states "Because the endocrine system plays a critical role in normal growth, development, and reproduction, even small disturbances in endocrine function may have profound and lasting effects. This is especially true during highly sensitive prenatal periods, such that small changes in endocrine status may have delayed consequences that are evident much later in adult life or in a subsequent generation. Furthermore, the potential for synergistic effects from multiple contaminants exists. The seriousness of the endocrine-disrupter hypothesis and the many scientific uncertainties associated with the issue are sufficient to warrant a coordinated federal research effort" (Environmental Protection Agency 2014b).

A growing number of organizations like the Huntington Breast Cancer Action Coalition, Environmental Working Group, Food and Water Watch, Americans against Fracking, Stop the Frack Attack, Concerned Health Professionals of New York (led by Sandra Steingraber), Pennsylvania Alliance for Clean Water, and BCA have placed fracking on their agenda in the past year. BCA's campaign "Don't Frack with Our Health" centers on raising awareness about the practice of fracking and how it leads to health problems.

Specifically organizations like BCA are concerned with the way the process of fracking allows water contamination and air pollution to compromise the health of people who live in the vicinity. They are also concerned with the way fracking chemicals can possibly contaminate food supply through the use of polluted water (BCA 2014a). The BCA contends that fracking is dangerous and grossly underregulated. While there are an increasing number of anti-fracking organizations, few identify their mission and focus in terms of women's health. Yet, among breast cancer organizations we see more and more groups (BCA, BCF) tackling fracking as a key environmental and women's health issue. For example in states like North Dakota, domestic violence shelters cite the large influx of male migrant workers as shifting the social lives of residents and increasing rates of domestic violence. In 2014 the Department of Justice began investigating the correlation between fracking and domestic violence. However, fracking has yet to enter onto the agenda of many domestic violence organizations, women's rights groups, or reproductive justice organizations despite the growing evidence of higher incidence rates of domestic violence and reproductive health problems in communities where fracking is occurring. Although at the local level, domestic violence shelters are certainly aware of the correlation between increased violence against women in fracking communities the evidence does not yet exist to demonstrate a causal relationship, merely a correlational one.

Many environmental and anti-fracking organizations advocate the precautionary principle. The precautionary principle demands that government agencies such as the Environmental Protection Agency regulate and protect us from the potential for harm. Moreover, in the face of uncertainty government agencies should act with caution. The level of uncertainty regarding the health impact of fracking is significant. This makes the need for using the precautionary principle even more important. The environmental justice movement, ecofeminists, and larger environmental movements also embrace this view (Carson 1994; Steingraber 1997b). The Toxic Substances Control Act (TSCA) would also require that chemicals be reported and disclosed. The TSCA is thought to be ineffective and outdated. It was passed in 1976. It requires that evidence of harm be provided as opposed to the precautionary principle, which advocates a better-safe-than-sorry approach. The TSCA represents one of the many policy failures to address environmental health problems that result from chemicals and toxins in fracking practices.

Organizations like BCF are advocating for a federal law that requires disclosure of chemicals used in fracking. In response to the energy companies' use of nondisclosure agreements to ensure silence about the harms of fracking, a federal law requiring disclosure would create transparency. Transparency is an important first step in being able to assess the true threat that fracking is to our health. Organizations like the BCF and the BCA support the Fracturing Responsibility and Awareness of Chemicals Act sponsored by Representative Diana DeGette (D-CO) and Senator Robert Casey (D-PA). The FRAC Act proposed by Congresspersons Jared Polis, Diana DeGette, and Maurice Hinchey tries to undo the hydraulic fracturing exemption from the Safe Drinking Water Act by requiring disclosure of chemicals.

In other words, we are just beginning to see the impact fracking is having on cancer incidence and advocates are working on multiple levels to achieve policy that bans fracking, research that investigates the links between fracking and breast cancer, and the model that encourages community-based participatory research. Government agencies like the Environmental Protection Agency are aware of the risk fracking poses to people's health and cancer risk yet the precautionary principle is not being used and instead people's health is at risk and the cancer burden is yet to be known in communities impacted by fracking. Despite this uncertainty, advocates are attacking this issue on multiple levels through both using citizen–science alliances and aiming to influence policy.

A Policy Focus

A number of studies try to explain why breast cancer gained the visibility that it did, and the changes in policy that followed. For example, Lerner (2001) examined the history of medical responses to breast cancer and its effect on women. On the basis of over 50 interviews with patients, survivors, and doctors, she followed the use of mammography and treatment options like radical mastectomy. She traced how decisions were made to pursue particular treatments and preventative measures. In addition, she provided a detailed historical account of the emergence of breast cancer as a public and political issue. Casamayou's *Politics of Breast Cancer* (2001) also tried to understand why breast cancer rose to the level of national policy in the late 1980s. She takes the spike in research funding as denoting a significant policy shift, and identifies new political players such as the NBCC as key to that development. She attributes the visibility and policy changes attributed to breast cancer advocacy as the result of a "triple alliance," defined as "protective congressional representatives with important committee posts, skillful executive agency personnel, and aggressive and resourceful interest groups and supporters" (Casamayou 2001: 32). Casamayou's important work is an early example of scholarship that sees organizations like NBCC as crucial to shaping the breast cancer movement, but her work does not focus on environmental prevention or look in depth at organization attributes. Organizations like Susan G. Komen for the Cure see themselves as helping move certain pieces of legislation forward. In fact, an advocate of the Massachusetts chapter of Komen sees the mission as ensuring its base has an understanding of relevant legislation and how it will affect women's lives and their treatment.

One of the NBCC's primary strategies is to lobby legislators to "end the breast cancer epidemic." As part of its Annual Advocacy Conference it trains participants in policy-making practices and strategies to influence public policy. The NBCC proposed "The Accelerating the End of Breast Cancer Act" and it is also fighting to ensure laws such as the "Patient Protection and Affordable Care Act" and Medicaid programs for cancer treatment are not repealed. There is some overlap in the type of policies that green and pink organizations will pursue. Because one of NBCC's tactics is to lobby politicians for specific legislation, it holds an annual conference dedicated to training advocates in political lobbying and to keep advocates informed of the most up-to-date medical perspectives on breast cancer. This model of policy reform, prevention-based knowledge dissemination, and advocacy training in scientific expertise seems to be the primary model for advocacy organizations such as the BCF and the NBCC.

The TSCA is thought to be ineffective and outdated as it was passed in 1976 and is in great need of reform. It requires that evidence of harm be provided as opposed to the precautionary principle, which advocates a better-safe-than-sorry approach. In fact, NBCC and BCF support the Reform of the Toxic Substances Control Act. A staff member at the MBCC states,

> We work on policy issues both on the state federal level and throughout the month of October and throughout the year, you know we try to mobilize our members to take action and to support change at the policy level. Specifically at the federal level we are focused on right now on a couple of bills such as The Safe Cosmetics Act and Reform of the Toxic Substances Control Act. So we are supporting efforts to put in place a structure in

which the government can take action on the most toxic chemicals and the link to health concerns like breast cancer and feel that companies need to be more forth coming about safety data and information.[18]

The TSCA represents one of the many policy failures to address environmental health problems that result from chemicals and toxins in fracking practices.

On the federal level, the NBCC and the MBCC, BCF, and BCA are supporting the Safe Chemicals Act, the Safe Cosmetics Act, and the Ban Poisonous Additives Act (BPA Ban Bill). The BCF supports more legislation relevant to environmental issues such as safe water, fracking, and pesticide use. We can see that these organizations primarily support legislation that has a cancer prevention–based environmental focus. This is in contrast to the policy solutions the Komen Foundation endorses. For example, the Susan G. Komen Foundation is currently seeking to approve the Breast Cancer Research Stamp authorization and the Breast Cancer Bill of Rights. The policy Susan G. Komen is working on fits within its focus on early detection and awareness. Despite its move toward more environmental research, its policy focus remains centered on the "pink" approach to breast cancer as opposed to one of prevention.

In conclusion, the results reported in this chapter demonstrate that the relationships among breast cancer advocacy organizations are highly interconnected. Many organizations seek the benefits of coalitions and networks while still maintaining their niche in the larger breast cancer movement. Key strategies among breast cancer advocates are to democratize science, build citizen–science alliances, and translate and disseminate scientific information. This is often done through the use of online tools such as Webinars, action alerts, and social networking. In addition, many organizations play a key role in advocating for legislation relevant to breast cancer at the state and federal levels.

Notes

1. Notes from speech by Joy Simha, NBCC Advocacy Training, Washington, DC, May 2011; in author's possession.

2. Anonymous, confidential interview by author, San Rafael, CA, February 10, 2011; in author's possession.

3. Anonymous, confidential interview by author, San Rafael, CA, February 10, 2011; in author's possession.

4. Anonymous, confidential interview by author, Boston, MA, November 16, 2010; in author's possession.

5. Anonymous, confidential phone interview by author, May 11, 2011; in author's possession.

6. Anonymous, confidential interview by author, San Rafael, CA, February 10, 2011; in author's possession.

7. Notes for Dr. Julia Brody's speech, NBCC Advocacy Training, Washington, DC, May 2011; in author's possession.

8. Activists in this area belonging to several organizations such as BCA, Greenpeace, Women's Cancer Resource Center, and West County Toxics Coalition formed the Toxic Links Coalition (Conrad and Leiter 2003:175).

9. Anonymous, confidential interview by author, San Francisco, CA, February 10, 2011, in author's possession.

10. Anonymous, confidential phone interview by author, May 11, 2011; in author's possession.

11. Anonymous, confidential phone interview by author, December 17, 2010; in author's possession.

12. Anonymous, confidential interview by author, San Rafael, CA, February 10, 2011; in author's possession.

13. Anonymous, confidential interview by author, Palo Alto, CA, February 11, 2011; in author's possession.

14. Anonymous, confidential interview by author, Palo Alto, CA, February 11, 2011; in author's possession.

15. Notes for Dr. Susan Love's speech, NBCC Advocacy Training, Washington, DC, May 2011; in author's possession.

16. Anonymous, confidential interview by author, San Rafael, CA, February 10, 2011; in author's possession.

17. BCA and other breast cancer organizations are also concerned about energy companies' pinkwashing. Companies like Chesapeake Energy (the parent company of Nomac Drilling) have been targeted by organizations like BCA for pinkwashing (BCA 2014c). This will be discussed further in Chapter 4.

18. Anonymous, confidential interview by author, Boston, MA, November 2011; in author's possession.

CHAPTER 4

Pink Ribbon Politics

An oncology nurse and patient advocate at Tufts Hospital states,

> Pink ribbons are actually tough because some people really embrace that and love it, and others want to throw up and say "I don't get that. I don't want to be associated with it." I have a number of breast cancer survivors who really hate pink—hate pink ribbons, hate October because it's Breast Cancer Awareness Month and they're going to see pink ribbons everywhere. You have to be sensitive to that. There are others who are very empowered by the camaraderie and the feeling cared for and enveloped into a community they never wanted to be invited to, but feel very supported by that.[1]

The oncology nurse's comments remind us that some survivors are drawn to the pink ribbon as it has come to symbolize hope, awareness, and support. The pink ribbon has come to be synonymous with breast cancer. The ubiquitous pink ribbon is a visible reminder of the success of breast cancer advocacy. The pink ribbon is everywhere on pens, mixers, mustangs, and candy, for example. In fact, the American public is bombarded with images of pink ribbons, requests for donations, action alerts, and publicized declarations of women's experiences of breast cancer. The success of the pink aspect of the movement is the ability to move this disease from isolation and shame into the public spotlight toward awareness and support. Yet, the pink ribbon continues to be polarizing and while for many it is a symbol of hope and a story of survivors, there are also those who see the pink ribbon as a reminder of the unfairness of the disease and the commercialization of the disease. For these people, the pink ribbon represents something problematic and controversial, or as Leopold (1999) refers to it, the dark side of the ribbon. For critics of the pink ribbon, it represents a type of advocacy that has ignored the relationship between environmental pollution and cancer. For these advocates, the search is not for a cure but rather for prevention and the pink ribbon is not only contentious but also toxic to women's health. Moreover, the use of the pink ribbon for a consumer-based activism has come to represent a corruption of the movement for some.

The Breast Cancer Action (BCA) often points out that the history of the pink ribbon is a history of pinkwashing and corporate influence over breast cancer advocacy. "Pinkwashing" refers to the corporate practice of using pink ribbons to sell products, which are linked to causing cancer (BCA 2010). In the early 1990s, a 68-year-old woman named Charlotte Haley, who was alarmed by the number of breast cancer diagnoses in her immediate family, attached peach-colored ribbons to postcards and distributed them to everyone she knew. The postcards read "The Nat'l Cancer Institute's annual budget is $1.8 billion, only 5 percent goes for cancer prevention. Help us wake up our legislators and America by wearing this ribbon" (BCA 2010). *Self* magazine and Estée Lauder cosmetics had heard about her ribbons and asked permission to use them as a promotional tool during National Breast Cancer Awareness Month (NBCAM). Haley refused because it was too commercial for her. *Self* and Estée Lauder consulted lawyers, who told them to change the color and it would be acceptable to use the ribbon without Haley's permission. *Self* and Estée Lauder held focus groups, which found that pink was soothing, comforting, and quieting, and the pink ribbon was born. Estée Lauder distributed millions of pink ribbons that year. Unfortunately, Charlotte Haley's message about cancer prevention is all too often lost among all the pink ribbons. It is worth remembering that this early message of prevention was discarded for the awareness and detection message being promoted by the founders of NBCAM.

As Chapter 3 discussed, the early days of the breast cancer movement were focused on spreading awareness and raising funds for research. In "Pink!: Community, Contestation, and the Color of Breast Cancer," Charlene Elliott states "Bathing our landscapes in pink is lovely, but it does not demand change: pink does not force corporations to account for the realities of a toxic environment that causes cancer; pink does not challenge medical procedures that disfigure women … pink does not question government policies" (Elliott 2007: 529). Elliott contends that pink is not contentious and arguably she is right; the pink ribbon, in the views of some advocates, makes the movement complicit with corporations who profit off of cancer and do not remove harmful chemicals from products.

Initially, many understood the pink ribbon to mean support of breast cancer movement and finding a cure. Although this remains largely true today, the pink ribbon has also been found more and more on consumer products that are best described as pink products. One can go into your average grocery store, mall, and bookstore and retail shops and most likely find some product for sale with a pink ribbon on it. The implication is that some portion of the proceeds will go toward breast cancer research. Upon closer examination of pink products it is revealed that often only a small portion of the sales are donated to breast cancer organizations and these donations tend to fund research on the pink agenda like lifestyle factors. However, very few people question how much money is donated, what specific foundations and organizations the money is donated to, or what research is supported. Although perhaps some corporations sell pink products to be responsible corporate citizens, it cannot be ignored that most companies stand to profit from this marketing strategy. The pink ribbon may mask a corporation's true motive of profit.

The practice of corporations using pink ribbons to sell products has become more and more common, starting in the late 1990s. It is clear that corporations wish to use the pink ribbons because it will increase sales and profitability. Scholars such as McCormick (2009), Ley (2009), and King (2008) have argued that the political economy of disease has shaped the breast cancer movement's overwhelming focus on the cure, treatment, support, and early detection. McCormick stated, "Political economy refers to the interrelationship between industry, our market-based economic system, and political institutions" (2009: 3). As a result of the political economy of breast cancer, at times corporate interests might prioritize profit over the pursuit of health. For example, corporations like General Electric (GE) profit tremendously from detection technology, such as mammography, and research for the cure whereas there is little profit in cancer prevention. McCormick stated, "In total, mammography usage is estimated to cost $5 billion to $13 billion per year (2009: 15). The revenue goes to companies that manufacture machines, technicians who provide the service, and hospitals that offer space where exams are conducted" (McCormick 2009: 15). Breast cancer is providing a very lucrative business for companies like GE. GE is a corporate sponsor of the

Susan G. Komen for the Cure and also the manufacturer of mammography machines. In fact, the pink aspect of the movement has capitalized on this brand of consumer activism to raise enormous amounts of funds for breast cancer research and raise awareness about the disease. Samantha King in *Pink Ribbons Inc.* has aptly documented and critiqued the problems with pink ribbons and consumer-based activism. King positions this type of activism and the use of corporate partnerships as a pink strategy, yet my findings indicate that both pink and green use corporate partnerships and at times consumer activism, but they use them in different ways. My findings also indicate that this issue of corporate involvement in advocacy is highly contentious among organizations and within the larger movement. For example, a program associate at BCA states,

> But I think that corporations know very well, I mean they are very, very focused on branding and image, obviously, because that's how they make money. That's how they stay in consumer's minds. It's huge for them. And they know very well that sort of issues tug at the heartstrings. Breast cancer is one of them, not just because people are, a lot of people are touched by breast cancer obviously but because breast cancer has been so linked with the feminine like pink and disquieting and it's just like this pleasant image which is peculiar. But anyway, but they know that linking their corporation, their name with a cause even if it's not breast cancer will appear to the consumers as if they're great even if they're Chevron or you know. And more than that, I mean I think the really insidious part of that is when they're pink washing.[2]

As the program associate points out many people are touched by breast cancer and emotionally moved when they see pink ribbons. As she points out, the pink ribbon is associated with a sentimentality and desire to support women with the disease that corporations capitalize on when they put pink ribbons on their products.

Corporations often promise to donate a portion of the proceeds to the breast cancer organization or vaguely to breast cancer research. For example, the Dansko shoe company sold pink ribbon clogs in 2010 where consumers likely believed a portion of profits were donated to breast cancer organizations. Yet, in this case Dansko agreed to pay a set amount of money in the sum of $25,000 to the Susan G. Komen Foundation (BCA 2012). The donation was the same and in this case Dansko was only obligated to donate the $25,000 regardless of the number of shoes sold. Capping the donation is a common practice. BCA who sees itself as the watchdog of the breast cancer movement uses its campaign "Think before You Pink" to expose egregious examples like Dansko. Yoplait yogurt owned by General Mills partnered with the Komen Foundation for its "Save Lids to Save Lives" campaign, which accounts for $1.1 billion of GM's "$11.2 billion in sales" (BCA 2012). In 1998, Yoplait teamed with Komen for the "Save Lids to Save Lives" campaign. In this campaign consumers bought the yogurt and sent in the lids where Yoplait makes a donation of 10 cents per lid, guaranteeing a minimum donation of $500,000, and a cap of $1.5 million (BCA 2012). The BCA critiques the Yoplait's campaign and informs us that one would have to eat three containers of Yoplait yogurt a day for four months to raise $36 for the Komen Foundation. Moreover, BCA's concern was that the dairy contained a bovine growth hormone linked to cancer. Examples such as Yoplait, Dansko, and numerous other examples demonstrate that corporations often set caps on their donations. This form of consumer-based activism is the primary strategy for fund-raising adopted by the pink aspect of the movement. It is also concerning that in some cases it is not clear which breast cancer organization is receiving the funds.

Arguably, this strategy of shopping our way out of the disease is the most controversial aspect of pink (King 2008). Samantha King, author of *Pink Ribbons, Inc.*, argues that the Susan G. Komen Foundation has successfully turned the disease into a marketable product and sees the breast cancer movement as a consumer-oriented philanthropic solution to social problems. BCA is concerned about the overwhelming number of products with a pink ribbon. Ultimately, one of its concerns is that the ingredients on many of these products are linked to causing cancer. It views many corporations as profiting off of cancer. BCA as an organization seeks to identify and publicly shame corporations who are "pinkwashers"; in other words organizations that profit from breast cancer. It coined this term "pinkwasher" as "a company that purports to care about breast cancer by promoting a pink ribbon campaign, but manufactures products that are linked to the disease" (BCA 2010). BCA's campaign "Think before You Pink" has identified Kentucky Fried Chicken, Yoplait, and many others as "pinkwashers." Take for example BCA's recent campaign against Kentucky Fried Chicken. Kentucky Fried Chicken ran a promotion "Buckets for the Cure," which encouraged people to buy fried chicken, and promised that a portion of the proceeds would be donated to the Komen Foundation. BCA critiqued this strategy as encouraging unhealthy choices for women, increasing profits for Kentucky Fried Chicken, while claiming to be concerned with breast cancer. Komen in a formal response to BCA defended its decision to work with Kentucky Fried Chicken as a way to reach millions of women and increase awareness about breast cancer. While the Kentucky Fried Chicken campaign could potentially have raised awareness for millions of women, BCA argues that it promotes an unhealthy diet, which is harmful to health. Komen's partnership with Kentucky Fried Chicken was criticized by multiple organizations. For example, a policy coordinator at Breast Cancer Fund (BCF) states,

But I'm not sure I want the profits of pharmaceutical companies being a major driving force within how people practice medicine. Not to put too fine a point on it, but when you have campaigns where you have pink ribbons on buckets of Kentucky Fried Chicken, you've gotta take a step back and say is that really the message we want to send. By eating Kentucky Fried Chicken, you're supporting breast cancer research? I think those kinds of things raise that question of what is the accountability that the organizations have to their missions and how do those corporate dollars influence or skew that.[3]

If corporate partnerships are meant to raise awareness, then campaigns like the Kentucky Fried Chicken's "Buckets for a Cure" are not problematic in and of itself. The Buckets for a Cure campaign and its use of the pink ribbon limit the larger movement to only one aspect, awareness. In this sense the pink ribbon and campaigns like "Buckets for a Cure" are not contentious enough, and do not align with the growing paradigm shift toward prevention, which sees cancer risk as eating healthy and reducing exposure to harmful hormones and toxins that might be found in fast food.

A Zero Breast Cancer staff member states,

So there was an example of a breast cancer organization last year who had advocated for breast cancer reductions and stuff but then prepared a label on KFC chicken wing container. That doesn't align with any breast cancer risk reduction message or any breast cancer prevention method. So I don't agree with that.[4]

Pink products and their perceived benefits or drawbacks were a key issue among the respondents. There was a varied response regarding the purchase of pink products. Although some respondents mentioned that pink products were problematic and even unethical, an equal number of people felt pink products were useful; even if it was a small portion of the proceeds going to cancer research, some respondents felt that this was better than nothing. Take a volunteer for Susan Love's Army of Women. She commented on buying pink products and seeing it as useful:

> Overall it is positive, if I get this product with a pink ribbon, then I thought about breast cancer critics saying it is only two cents to the cause. But it is two cents that wouldn't have otherwise gone to breast cancer advocacy.[5]

She followed up these comments by emphasizing the need for corporations who sell pink products to be transparent and accountable for how much money is going to breast cancer. Similarly, a Susan G. Komen staff member when asked about corporate giving campaigns states,

> It has to be um a really complementary piece in regards to our strategic planning. That yes we heavily depend on the dollars in order to support programming at the local level but that is not the sole purpose. That there are these different facets and that they all have to align with one another to insure that we are getting to the root of the issue and more importantly fulfilling our mission as an organization.[6]

Almost all respondents suggested there needs to be better accountability standards to regulate corporate partnerships with organizations, meaning that this is a virtue that members and staff of both pink and green value.

The National Breast Cancer Coalition's (NBCC) campaign "Breast Cancer Deadline 2020" calls attention to the failures of the breast cancer movement and the pink ribbon. Fran Visco, president of NBCC, in a fund-raising mailer sent out in 2012 stated:

> It is unacceptable that at a time when pink ribbons adorn everything from cereal boxes to baseball caps to billboards that so little actual progress has been made toward ending breast cancer.

How can it be that in a country that devotes so much attention and resources to breast cancer, breast cancer incidence and mortality have not budged significantly in decades? In fact, in the U.S., the chance of a woman developing breast cancer in her lifetime has actually *increased* from about 1 in 11 in 1975 to 1 in 8 today (Visco 2012).

Pink products have been successful at raising funds but less successful at reducing breast cancer incidence. In other words, it is not clear that pink ribbons are reducing breast cancer and this is why the green organizations' tendency to critique pink ribbons often goes hand in hand with a message of prevention. Visco is asking members to donate funds but also to urge President Obama to endorse the Breast Cancer Deadline 2020. NBCC sees political support as crucial to the success of this campaign and the prevention of breast cancer, and wants much more than pink ribbons, which focus on awareness and early detection.

The BCF and the BCA have specific organizational rules and policies regarding funding. The rules are meant to prevent corporate influence over advocacy strategies and action. Green organizations such as BCA have been known to critique pink organizations such as Komen regarding corporate influence over advocacy, yet the findings of this research indicate that all organizations, both pink and green, establish rules and norms regarding corporate donations and sponsorships. Although the majority of this book has been aimed at demonstrating the way pink and green organizations are converging along the notion of prevention, this chapter presents a key difference that remains among pink and green organizations. The remaining divide between pink and green is regarding consumer activism, pink products, and corporate partnerships. However, advocacy relationships with corporations are often met with deep suspicion and concern about undue influence over an organization's actions. Corporate giving campaigns and consumer activism are controversial for the breast cancer movement.

Many advocates express concern about where the money from fund-raising goes and what types of corporations are donating to the cause of breast cancer. Advocates desire transparency about fundraising proceeds. Several members of pink organizations mentioned that prior to getting involved, they researched both Susan G. Komen and the Avon foundations to examine where the fund-raising money goes and what portion actually goes to the cause as opposed to the organization itself, and how much money was distributed locally.

It is clear from the qualitative interviews performed that participants in the breast cancer movement are quite informed and concerned about transparency within advocacy organizations.

Circle of Profit

BCA identifies a "cancer profit circle," which refers to when corporations help cause cancer and then sell cancer treatments and drugs (BCA 2012). This circle of profit is an interesting concept to understand breast cancer culture. I would argue that this conceptual framework could be expanded. A circle of profit framework can also help us understand when corporations create products linked to causing cancer and then donate significant portions of money to cancer research. Many corporations such as GE and drug companies stand to profit from the movement's focus on treatment and early detection. McCormick (2009) cited AstraZeneca as an example of a corporation that manufactures breast cancer drugs, which bring in $19 billion a year. AstraZeneca also owns the rights to and is the main corporate sponsor of NBCAM (McCormick 2009). The case of AstraZeneca has been widely documented by breast cancer scholars (Klawiter 2008; Ley 2009; McCormick 2009) as deeply troubling. Another example is the Avon Foundation's production of cosmetics with carcinogens, which bring in enormous profit, while simultaneously Avon is a public face of breast cancer advocacy and one of breast cancer research's larger donors. The Campaign for Safe Cosmetics has asked Avon to sign the Campaign for Safe Cosmetics where Avon would pledge to remove chemicals linked to causing cancer from its products, and Avon is yet to sign this pledge. In fact, the Campaign for Safe Cosmetics is organizationally tied to the BCF, and both have accused Avon of pinkwashing. McCormick stated,

> For example, Avon raises funds for breast cancer through its Cosmetics for the Cure and Kiss Breast Cancer Good-Bye cause-marketing campaigns. Proceeds from these promotions contribute to the company's $350 million global total for fundraising as of 2004. Ironically, one of the products that Avon sells for its campaign is laden with potentially carcinogenic chemicals. (2009: 131)

Groups like the Safe Cosmetics Alliance and the Environmental Working Group have called attention to Avon's problematic relationship with cancer and pointed out the various ingredients in its cosmetics that are very harmful. If we understand this circle of profit framework, it becomes quite clear that the link between corporations and breast cancer advocacy can be quite problematic. One participant who has worked on the Safe Cosmetics Campaign and the Alliance for Health Tomorrow offers her perspective on the link between consumer-based activism, corporations, and advocacy. At the time of the interview a Boston resident, she described seeing the Avon walkers and being frustrated with the pink message and Avon's use of pinkwashing:

> I think there is always a risk in having corporate involvement because so many of these corporations are producing chemicals that cause cancer and then are producing the drugs that treat cancer. That to me is the biggest problem. I don't see corporate giving necessarily as a problem in and of itself but I think in the way, the corporations that are making the most money off of this I observe as the biggest problem ... I think that the biggest problem from a public engagement, social movement perspective is that [consumer activism] is giving people a sort of false sense of security. I've bought this thing, I've done my part for this and I've done something about breast cancer and that's a problem. It is a sort of shifting tension away from the actual issue. Potato chips (that have a pink ribbon) have nothing to do with breast cancer.[7]

She is concerned that purchasing pink ribbon products can be harmful to one's health if you are ingesting toxic chemicals but also that it may lead to a type of political apathy that displaces attention away from preventing breast cancer. In fact Susan G. Komen's Promise Me perfume was found to contain unhealthy ingredients not listed on the packaging. Unlisted chemicals in Promise Me perfume that are known to be toxic and hazardous include Galaxolide, which works as a hormone disruptor, and Toluene, a neurotoxicant linked to negative health effects. Toluene is even banned by the International Fragrance Association and yet it was present in Susan G. Komen's perfume where the sales proceeds went to breast cancer research. Post World War II there has been a chemical boom but testing and regulation have not been adequate. For example, out of the 100,000 chemicals registered for market use, health data are only available for less than 10% (BCA 2012).

Corporate Partnerships

At times corporations choose to sponsor or partner with breast cancer organizations. Many of the breast cancer organizations are concerned about corporate influence on research and advocacy. Their concern is a result of the sometimes inappropriate corporate relations between breast cancer advocacy and research. In breast cancer advocacy, many organizations rely on corporate sponsorships. King (2008) traces the more prevalent corporate strategy of sponsorships of breast cancer organization. She cites Bristol-Myers Squibb, Estée Lauder, Ford, GE, and the NFL as just some examples of breast cancer consumer philanthropy (2008: 1–2). The Komen Foundation identifies 22 corporate sponsors who have donated at least $1 million and who are devoted to the cause as the Million Dollar Council. These corporate sponsors include Bristol-Myers Squibb, BMW, American Airlines, KitchenAid, and Payless. Corporate sponsors such as Bristol-Myers Squibb who is a leading pharmaceutical distributor highlight the fact that breast cancer has become a marketable issue and an opportunity for big businesses to demonstrate their philanthropic side. King (2008) stated, "companies and brands associate themselves with a cause as a means to build the reputation of a brand, increase profit, develop employee loyalty to the company, and add to their reputation as good corporate citizens" (King 2008: 9). In other words corporations stand to profit when they associate themselves with a charitable cause like breast cancer research. King (2008) and BCA also identify Susan G. Komen's use of corporate sponsors as particularly problematic. Susan G. Komen is not alone in utilizing corporate sponsorships to pursue activist goals. The Avon Foundation and BCF also use corporate partnerships to pursue their goals. It has been an increasingly common strategy in breast cancer advocacy to use corporate partners and for these corporations to employ pink product marketing, which will be discussed in the following section.

Susan G. Komen Foundation events such as "Race for the Cure" are the most obvious example of the role corporate sponsors plays in breast cancer advocacy. Attending a "Race for the Cure," one is inundated with corporate logos, advertising, and promotional speeches. One also receives "freebies" such as Yoplait yogurt, Ford paraphernalia, and T-shirts listing the corporate sponsors. Ley (2009) reported that the largest portion of Susan G. Komen's budget comes from corporate partners. Yet former CEO of Komen reports that corporate influence over the board's decisions is not likely. Ultimately, some advocates are concerned that corporations will have undue influence over an organization's strategies and missions. Former CEO of the Komen Foundation who has sat on multiple boards at various cancer advocacy organizations disagreed. She suggested that individual wealthy donors who sit on boards have more potential to influence an organization negatively than a corporation. She argued that, in practice, corporate giving campaigns were more hands-off than funds that came from government or even private donors.

> It is interesting, in most cases and in my experience with corporate giving campaigns, it is more hands off and restricted than funds that come from government or private donors. There is more potential for influence from other sources of funds granted. There are some cases when an organization takes funds with no guidelines. The more careful organizations do not take from corporations that would try to influence them. Wealthy donors will ask to sit on boards and that person can try to call the shots. This has more potential for damage. We should not be so concerned about corporate funds and vilify corporate funds and put a halo on individual donors. In my twenty years, only once has a corporation asked for a seat on the board. It is individual donors who want that seat on the board. I believe we all act out of goodness and the best intentions but sometimes this can go wrong, but if we create such clear strategies and rules about who can do what. . .[8]

As this participant shows rules about who can do what might prevent individual donors from being able to influence a board of directors. This suggests that while there is great concern about corporate influence on advocacy organizations, it is not clear that this has actually occurred in practice as often. Interviews with board members do demonstrate their significant potential to shape the mission and strategy of their organization. For example, Zero Breast Cancer discussed its decision to accept funds from Avon and how it has not tried to influence them in any way. According to a board member there,

> We do accept money from the Avon Foundation, and that was a big issue with the organization. Oh, in many, many, board meetings we were really kind of unsure of how much they would influence or how much influence they would exert on us in terms of what we were doing, or what research we participated in.

But we . . . also everyone at the table decided it would be a teach-able moment for Avon. We would take this money and of course the reason they gave it to us was a direct result of Barbara Brenner having initiated her campaign against Avon, saying that they need to run the walk themselves, and be very transparent about how they return the money to the community. So actually Avon contacted us and asked us if we were interested . . . I mean never once have I have ever had any communication between or any message that we needed to do anything . . . .[9]

As the board member states, Avon was donating money to environ-mental organizations like Zero Breast Cancer with no strings attached; in this sense there was no undue influence as is sometimes suspected. Concerns about corporate influence extended to concerns that when major organizations like Susan G. Komen and Avon fund smaller organ-izations there might be an agenda that would compromise a focus on prevention. Yet as we can see with the case of Avon and Zero Breast Cancer, this has not been the case. Avon also provides funding for the Silent Spring Institute and this is evidence of Avon's increasing willing-ness to consider environmental links to cancer, as it is funding organiza-tions whose main purpose is to extrapolate this link.

Corporate philanthropy, pink ribbon products, and the corporate partnerships have been staples of breast cancer advocacy. The findings of this research demonstrate that despite caution, there is a growing consensus that relationships with corporations can be mutually benefi-cial. A Zero Breast Cancer staff member states,

I think as long as it aligns with what you're doing that that's great. And I think I also believe in social entrepreneurship and social responsibility as part of corporations. So as long as it aligns with they're doing and doesn't contradict their mission, then I think it's fine.[10]

Consensus-based decision-making processes would hopefully prevent one individual from exerting too much influence over a board; how-ever it is equally possible that individuals just as much as corporations can influence organizations for their own agenda. BCF, BCA, Zero Breast Cancer, all described their decision-making process as consen-sus based.

Although the BCF uses corporate partners to pursue its goals, it is different in important ways. Organizations like the BCF emphasized their strict guidelines regarding corporate donations. For example, the BCF has a very strong public relationship with Luna because this corporation has similar mission, style, and principles. It also maintains relationships with Seventh Generation (a company that manufactures green cleaning products) and feels that with careful examination there is a place for corporate funding, according to a seasoned advocate and board member at the BCF. Therefore, organizations like BCF maintain that there is a place in breast cancer advocacy for corporate giving campaigns.

The process of deciding to work with like-minded companies should be carefully considered. A policy coordinator at BCF states,

> We do partner with like-minded companies. So any company that is interested in working with us, we go through a very intense vetting process to make sure that they have the same values as we do as well as not producing products or anything that is toxic to health and the environment. Because we think it's about a full cycle as well. It's not just is your product safe? It's are your manufacturing process safe?[11]

Organizations like BCF assess a potential partner by its commitment to toxic-free products and as such BCF has partnered with companies like Klean Kanteen and Luna Bars.

The program coordinator at BCF also states,

> I have a real problem with people selling pink products just to get on the bandwagon and selling products that are full of toxic chemicals, let's say. You can't be part of the problem and purport to be part of the solution in the same breath and really come across as having a lot of integrity. But I think that companies who are truly committed to the work—and we work with some of them who are really creating viable alternatives to solve these issues and who are very open to a two-way conversation—that they really want to partner with organizations whose missions mesh.[12]

However, this differs remarkably from organizations like the BCA who pride themselves on refusing almost all corporate donations (only 2% of BCA's revenue comes from corporate funding; BCA, 2015d). BCA sees itself as quite distinct from other advocacy organizations precisely because it takes a hard and clear line on "pinkwashing."

According to BCA's Web site it refuses to take contributions from anyone that it views as profiting from breast cancer. Currently 74% of its funding comes from individual donations. When an individual donates, if his or her employer is part of a donation-matching program, BCA will accept the funds. Theoretically, if an individual from Chevron donated to BCA through a matching program, the donation would be accepted, despite the fact that BCA is opposed to taking a corporate donation from Chevron. Some companies like Chevron agree to match a dollar amount that employees make for donations to certain charities and organizations. Staff member of BCA stated, "We accept matching programs if someone works for Chevron—and if that individual chooses to make a donation, we will accept." However, it is explicitly against profiting from the cancer industry. This policy of refusing to accept money from anyone who profits from cancer or contributes to pollution emerged out of a controversy in 1998 where Chevron had donated money to the BCF. According to Brenner "As a result of that controversy, Sandra Steingraber wrote a letter to the Fund, which she shared with me, explaining her view that silence is the sound of money talking. That controversy prompted BCA to take another look at corporate contributions. The board ultimately adopted a written policy rejecting any funding from companies or entities that were profiting from cancer or contributing to the polluting of the environment" (Brenner 2012, oral history by Pluss, 16). BCA argues, ultimately this organizational rule is responsible for its freedom to voice concerns of activist tactics and its credibility to question certain organizations and corporations. Specifically, BCA will criticize other organizations like the Susan G. Komen for the Cure for partnering with GE or Chevron.

An examination of organizations' resources, funding, and policies on corporate partnerships reveals key differences between pink and green organizations and their strategies. It is equally important to investigate how advocacy organizations are influenced by the corporations they work with, their funding sources, and their relationship to cause marketing. BCA argues that organizations are susceptible to be influenced by corporate partnerships. Interviews with staff indicate that BCA purposefully keeps a small staff of nine people so that the majority of its money goes toward funding its programs to support its mission. If we compare the resources of BCA, we will find a much different story. The BCA, for example, lists total revenue of $680,098 in 2010–2011. Individual contributions consist of 74% of its total revenue and corporate funding accounts only for 2% (BCA, 2012). A staff member, at BCA, stated:

We do not take money from anyone that contributes to or profits from breast cancer. There should be no profiteering from the cancer industry. It allows us to speak with credibility with issues about funding and what motivates certain organizations. Low and behold, Susan G. Komen has partnered with General Electric. How can you speak honestly and advocate in a non-partisan way for an ending of this disease, when you are partnering with a company for whom this disease is their bread and butter.[13]

The BCA serves as an example where it devotes the bulk of its resources to its strategic plans. Individuals primarily fund BCA whereas corporations like GE and fund-raising events like the race primarily fund the Komen foundation for the Cure.

A comparison to the national Susan G. Komen foundation reveals much larger budgets. According to Ley,

In fiscal year 2005–2006, Komen amassed a $268 million budget for its activities. Although the organization generated almost $15 million of this budget through "other public support and revenue," it garnered almost $120 million from the Race for the Cure series. It is contributions, however, that represent the largest portion of Komen's budget at $133 million. (2009: 127)

The largest funders of breast cancer research include National Cancer Institute, National Institute of Health, Department of Defense, Avon, Susan G. Komen, and the American Cancer Society, to name a few (McCormick 2009). Organizations such as Avon and Susan G. Komen that contribute the most are most likely to shape the research toward a biomedical research agenda. Events like Avon's Breast Cancer Crusade and the Susan G. Komen Foundation's Race for the Cure raise millions of dollars. Phil Brown in *Toxic Exposures* argued that federal breast cancer research has seen greater funding, yet "less than 3 percent of the money (a total of $800 million in 2001) has been directed toward finding environmental connections to breast cancer" (McCormick 2009: 187). Here we can clearly see the privileging of a biomedical research agenda as evidenced by less than 3% funding that goes toward environmental connections. Susan G. Komen has considerably larger resources than organizations like BCA and we see that its focus on medical research for the cure has dominated the cancer research agenda in the United States.

The Susan G. Komen Foundation, NBCC, and BCF demonstrated a nuanced view that corporate philanthropy was not bad in itself, but it is the way some corporations use the pink ribbon that is troubling. For example, a former member of the board of directors at the BCF describes BCF's view on corporate donations. She states:

> We take corporate money but we have strict guidelines. For example, we would never take money from Chevron. We don't appeal to them either. If an employee from Chevron wants to give and its matched, then fine. We have a strong partnership with Luna because that corporation matches our mission and style. It is a great relationship. We have just added a new company for sustainable products. We get a percentage for every shoe they sell. Some corporations are targeted by us to work with. For example, 7th Generation, but we would not ever seek out Clorox. We are very careful, so there is a place for corporate funding.[14]

Her statement and BCF's corporate partnerships demonstrate the view that corporate relationships are not always harmful or overly influential of an organization's mission or agenda. A policy coordinator at BCF states,

> Corporate giving campaigns can certainly be an important source of resources for a movement that needs that. We all do a lot with a little. But we could certainly do a lot more with more. And many of them do it for all the right reasons—many of the corporations. On the other hand, to the extent that giving money gives them a seal of approval while their other corporate practices undermine the very goals that we are seeking to achieve. Then it's that cross-purposes and influences the integrity of how advocacy organizations approach their work. It's a conversation we have a lot. It's an issue that I don't know that I would say it's so in the breast cancer world, although, potentially but certainly the pharmaceutical world has had enormous influence on the way medicine gets practiced in this country—for good or for worse.[15]

Pink ribbons have come to be associated with a consumer-based activism and breast cancer advocates from both pink and green articulate nuanced views about the role corporations should play in advocacy, the impact of pink ribbons and its association with awareness and detection as opposed to prevention.

The green movement organizations like BCA or BCF mostly receive funding from private donations. For example, BCA sees itself as quite distinct from other advocacy organizations precisely because it takes a hard and clear line on "pinkwashing." BCA refuses to take contributions from anyone that it views as profiting from breast cancer. Currently 74% of its funding comes from individual donations. However, some of the green organizations like the BCF take a more moderate approach and accept donations from "like minded" corporations.

In essence, this means that BCF only accepts donations from corporations that are committed to environmental concerns and cancer prevention. The concern is that corporations influence the organization's agenda and therefore the larger research agenda. The green movement differs remarkably on this matter of funding from the pink. For example, the largest portion of Susan G. Komen's budget comes from corporate partners. This is significant because the largest funders of breast cancer research include National Cancer Institute, National Institute of Health, Department of Defense, Avon, Susan G. Komen, and the American Cancer Society, to name a few (McCormick 2009). The role of corporations in health advocacy is an extremely contentious point in the movement, yet my research shows that Susan G. Komen has been influenced by individual political agendas of board members and corporations. Susan G. Komen has considerably larger resources than organizations like BCA and we see that Komen's focus on medical research for the cure has dominated the cancer research agenda in the United States. Ultimately, it seems like the concern is that corporations will have undue influence over advocacy strategies and missions.

Corporate Partnerships: The Case of Fracking

As discussed in Chapter 3, the links between fracking and environmental harm and health problems are alarming. Fracking exposes people to toxic chemicals of concern and some of these chemicals are linked to cancer. Moreover, the role fracking is playing in increasing breast cancer risk makes recent examples of Susan G. Komen's partnerships with a fracking company deeply concerning. Companies like Chesapeake Energy (the parent company of Nomac Drilling) have been targeted by organizations like BCA for pinkwashing (BCA 2014c). In celebration of breast cancer awareness, Nomac Drilling wrapped its drill rigs in pink in 2012. Similarly, Baker Hughes, an oil field service company and leader in the fracking industry, partnered with the Susan G. Komen Foundation during the NBCAM 2014 to circulate 1,000 pink drill bits and donated $100,000 (BCF 2015). Baker Hughes's campaign titled "Doing Our Bit for the Cure" is in its words "supporting research, screening, and education to help find the cures of the disease, which claims a life every 60 seconds" (Baker Hughes 2015). The check was presented to the Susan G. Komen Foundation on October 26, 2014, in Pittsburg at an NFL game. Baker Hughes also sponsors the Survivor Pin Celebration at the annual Houston Race for the Cure (Baker Hughes 2015). Susan G. Komen's partnership with Baker Hughes is a particularly egregious example of pinkwashing because Susan G. Komen acknowledges on its Web site that certain chemicals are associated with cancer risk. These same chemicals are also found in fracking fluid. The case of the pink drill bits serves as a reminder that while Susan G. Komen is increasingly moving toward a message of prevention and a recognition in environmental causes of cancer, partnerships with companies that contribute to cancer still remain.

Internal Dynamics and Decision Making

To understand why both pink and green organizations have shifted toward a message of environmental cancer prevention, one must first understand how decisions are made within these organizations. This book aims to make such a contribution by using qualitative data to demonstrate the shift toward prevention as a result of decision-making processes within the organizations. In *Advocacy Organizations and Collective Action*, edited by Prakash and Gugerty, author Maryann Barakso (2010) argued that it is important to examine the internal dynamics of advocacy organizations. This book extends Barakso's argument by showing the ways internal dynamics have played a key role in shaping the larger movement's direction toward prevention. I argue that as "green" organizations have become more professionalized, they have begun to mirror "pink" organizations with regard to their internal dynamics. This change in which green organizations appear similar to pink organizations helps us to understand the larger convergence between the two.

The results show that breast cancer organizations are often similar to bureaucracies in having clear rules, job descriptions, budgets, and offices, and that these factors inform strategy, which supports the social movement literature. A qualitative analysis of the interviews conducted for this study with staff and board members shows that organizations rely on rules and decision-making structures to act. To understand the decisions made by these advocacy organizations, we must first understand the conditions in which organizations make decisions, and this book aims to make such a contribution. In the context of breast cancer advocacy organizations, the qualitative interviews revealed traditional top-down decision-making or consensus-based decision-making practices are most commonly used. An analysis of the data shows that these organizations' boards of directors have played a key role in privileging a message of prevention and shaping the mission. Based on these findings, this chapter argues that a close examination of the characteristics of a few breast cancer organizations demonstrates patterns of structure and decision-making processes within them. The BCA and the Susan G. Komen Foundation are both national-level organizations. If we compare these organizations to the Susan G. Komen's national chapter, we see quite a difference in terms of staff, size, and resources.

The BCA, led by executive director Karuna Jaggar, currently has eleven members who sit on the board of directors and nine staff members whose positions focus on mobilization, communications, membership, and office services. They are also influenced by a Scientific Advisory Board and the National Advisory Council. The Scientific Advisory Board is made up primarily of PhDs, genetic counselors, public health officials, surgeons, oncologists, and academics, whereas their National Advisory Council is made up of leaders of other breast cancer advocacy organizations, authors, activists, and women's health advocates. Based on the findings of this research, BCA sees itself as creating programs and making decisions through committees with a consensus-based process. BCA staff member described the decision-making process as follows:

> In terms of decisions we make, we have a lot of committees. It is a lot of consensus. It is a constant struggle to flatten the organization versus hierarchize. I think we do a pretty good job of doing that. We ask who is marginal, who is marginalized? It really impacted the way we negotiate meetings. If you've got eight people, they are very opinionated, not necessarily opinionated but loud and savvy, there are age discrepancies from 18 to 63.[16]

Her views and other interviews with BCA participants show that the organization's goal is to promote consensus-based decision making and an active reflection on power dynamics within the organization.

In the qualitative interviews with members of several advocacy organizations, BCA's emphasis on consensus-based decision making was rather unique. I show that the majority of breast cancer advocacy organizations use a top-down approach and therefore the board of directors exerts considerable influence. A former CEO of the Komen Foundation, and who at the time of the interview was a director of Commonweal, an environmental health institute, is extremely experienced in breast cancer advocacy.[17] In addition to Commonweal and the Susan G. Komen for the Cure, she has also worked with the National Cancer Institute and the American Society of Cancer Oncology. She provided an experienced and nuanced view given her work with both the Susan G. Komen Foundation and an environmental institute like Commonweal. She claimed that the board of directors has the most influence over Susan G. Komen and that this has potential to shape organizational strategies that reflect individual agendas. In fact, she suggested that members of the board at any given organization have the potential to pursue their own agendas, which can be problematic. This could be more of a danger to an organization, because it would subject an organization's focus to the beliefs of individual agendas. Scholars such as King (2008) and organizations like BCA have argued that corporate sponsors have the greatest potential to influence an organization. However, the results of this research find it is not clear that an organization is more influenced by corporate sponsors and instead find that individual board members exert greater influence. The participant's assertion is compelling also because it reveals how important rules for decision-making processes are in an organization.

The potential for individual agendas to influence a board and therefore an organization's mission and strategy is great. This is most accurately seen in the recent controversy surrounding Susan G. Komen's initial defunding of Planned Parenthood. Susan G. Komen publicly received an enormous amount of criticism so much so that Susan G. Komen eventually reinstated the funds for Planned Parenthood to provide services to the medically underserved. In public statements, Susan G. Komen claimed that this was a decision made by the board of directors. Interestingly the *Atlantic* cites John Hammerly who served as a senior communications advisor for Susan G. Komen as describing a small group of individuals who had an agenda to defund Planned Parenthood due to its antiabortion beliefs. In the article Hammerly is quoted as saying "About a year ago, a small group of people got together inside the organization to talk about what the options were, what would be the ramifications of staying the course, or of telling our affiliates they can't fund Planned Parenthood, or something in between." He went on, "As we looked at the ramifications of ceasing all funding, we felt it would be worse from a practical standpoint, from a public-relations standpoint, and from a mission standpoint. The mission standpoint is, how could we abandon our commitment to the screening work done by Planned Parenthood? But the Susan G. Komen board made the decision despite the recommendation of the organization's professional staff to keep funding Planned Parenthood" (*Atlantic* 2012). As we can see from Hammerly's comments, there was a tension between fulfilling the organization's mission and fulfilling the personal agendas of a few select people on the board of directors at Komen. Komen initially claimed that one of the updated rules to their grant-making process required that they defund Planned Parenthood. That rule stated,

> Currently, a Komen grant may be terminated if, among other things, the grantee loses or changes its tax exempt status, is barred from receiving federal or state funds, or if we learn of any financial and/or administrative improprieties. Going forward, these same standards will now also be used in determining eligibility for Komen grants. (*Atlantic* 2012)

However, Hammerly insisted that the rule was created to allow Susan G. Komen to defund Planned Parenthood specifically. Ultimately, the public outcry against Susan G. Komen pressured it to reinterpret its rule and continue to fund Planned Parenthood. However, Mollie Williams was forced to resign from the Susan G. Komen board because it was perceived that her antiabortion politics is what was responsible for shaping Susan G. Komen's agenda. In other words, I argue there is concern about the decision-making processes and how much influence individuals' beliefs have in shaping an entire advocacy organization. Therefore this book extends King's scholarship on corporate influence in the breast cancer movement by presenting data that show board members and decision-making processes are influential as well.

Running, Walking, and Hiking in Pink

Physical endurance activities have become a primary strategy of both green and pink breast cancer advocacy organizations. Events where one might run, walk, swim, hike, kayak, or bike for a cure are very common today. These physical endurance events began with the Susan G. Komen's Race for the Cure. In 1983 Komen introduced physical fitness fund-raisers, what we know today as the Race for the Cure. Komen held its first race in 1983 in Dallas, Texas, and in 1990 held its first National Race for the Cure in Washington, DC. In 1990 Komen gave out pink visors to cancer survivors participating in the Race for the Cure and one year later was giving out pink ribbons to every participant in NYC races, and finally in 1992 became the symbol of NBCAM (Sulik 2012: 47). Komen also holds a 3-day, 60-mile walk in various cities across the United States, where an individual must raise a minimum of $2,300 to participate. Similarly the Avon Foundation holds a two-day event where an individual must raise a minimum of $1,800 to participate and walk 39.3 miles. Both Avon and Komen use a similar model of multiple-day walking events to fund-raise for breast cancer research.

King states

> Commodities such as the Race for the Cure (you pay in exchange for opportunity to participate, an official T-shirt, and "freebies" that vary with each race) also appear to illuminate or reveal the virtuosity of those who buy them, to transform purchasers into certain kinds of people living certain kinds of lives. Thus, the National Race for the Cure might be understood as a site for the production of both consumer-citizens and corporate citizens and as such exemplifies the ways in which citizenship advances through consumption at this particular moment in history. (King 2008: 39)

The Susan G. Komen Breast Cancer Foundation in 2004 invested $98.6 million in grants and programs for breast cancer research, education, screening, and treatment. The Komen Foundation spent 75 cents of every dollar raised on mission programs and services (Komen Foundation 2006).

Gayle Sulik in *Pink Ribbon Blues* has aptly argued the gendered and nationalist metaphors used to discuss breast cancer. Sulik offers an insightful analysis of the ways that pink ribbon has become steeped in gender discourse that positions femininity in traditional passive and docile ways. The pink ribbon as a symbol of breast cancer is also a symbol of the gendered expectations that correlate with the expectations society has of how women should deal with cancer. In this sense, the pink ribbon does more than represent a consumer-based model of advocacy but also reinscribes traditional gender norms.

Western society places an enormous emphasis on women's breasts as important parts of the body. In *Manmade Breast Cancers*, Zillah Eisenstein argues the breast is loaded with social meaning because it is a visible symbol of maternity, femininity, and sexual desire (Eisenstein 2001). In contemporary culture, women's breasts are understood as maternal, sexual, and/or objectified. In "Breasted Experience," Iris Young argues breasts convolute the boundaries of motherhood and sexuality (Young 2005). There is a tension in understanding women's breasts as both maternal and sexual. In the context of breast cancer, women's breasts and their bodies are also constructed as either maternal or sexual entities. The sexual breast and the maternal breast are considered to be an important part of women's feminine identity but in different ways.

In contemporary culture women's breasts are fetishized as a representation of feminine sexuality. Eve Kosofsky Sedgwick, in "Breast Cancer: An Adventure in Applied Deconstruction," argues that breast cancer while thought to challenge femininity does the exact opposite (Sedgwick 1999). Sedgwick argues breast cancer "plunges one into an experience of almost archetypal femininity" (Sedgwick 1999: 154). Breast cancer often can lead to removal of the breast and therefore has a tendency to lead women to both mourn and reconsider the source of their femininity. In Western society, breasts have become symbols of female sexuality and therefore breast cancer draws our attention to cultural understandings of what it means to be a woman.

In contrast to the sexual entity, women's breasts are also seen as giving life and nourishment to children. According to Samantha King in *Think Pink, Inc.*, breast cancer poses a threat to one of the major roles women play in society, which is mother (King 2008). It poses a threat because it can be a lethal disease that can prevent women from being mothers, and thereby depriving women of what is often considered to be their best contribution to society. Perhaps this fact is the cause of the enormous public engagement in breast cancer activism. Understanding the breast as maternal leads to a view of the breast as functional. In other words, the breast's primary purpose is to nourish babies. This understanding of the maternal breast as functional contributes to the objectification of breasts.

Young (2005) argues that women's breasts are constructed as objects. Young (2005) points out that Western medicine sees breasts as an object or a part of the body that can be dispensable. Similarly, Lerner argues that the breast is seen as useless unless a woman is pregnant (Lerner 2001: 88). Lerner (2001) provides comments made by physicians as evidence to the conception of the breast as nonvital. She cites George Pack who states "breasts in women unlikely to ever breast feed were 'useless.' " (Lerner 2001: 40). This physician's statement constructs women's bodies and their breasts only in terms of reproductive function and denies women's sexual relationship with their breasts, and it also presents women's breasts only in binary terms. This understanding of women's breasts as dispensable and not vital, historically, has led to recommendations of radical mastectomy when dealing with breast cancer. Yet society tells us just the opposite; women's breasts are indeed vital. The breast while perhaps not vital to life is vital to women's identity in contemporary culture. Therefore, while the breast does not play a vital role in sustaining women or children's lives, it clearly does play an important function socially. Otherwise reconstruction after mastectomy would not be so popular. There are countless narratives by women who have undergone mastectomy discussing the emotional loss of the breast and one's femininity. Because the breast is positioned in such a way, cancer and/or the removal of breasts threatens and reinforces women's identity as feminine sexual beings.

Young (2005) argues Western culture often conflates women's breasts with a woman's sense of self. Young (2005) argues it is not a surprise that many women have a difficult time with the loss of the breast because according to Young this is a loss of the self. Clearly the breast holds significance for women's sense of self. Despite this clear link between the breast, femininity, and a woman's sense of self, contemporary culture still thinks of women's breasts as objectified parts. When breasts are constructed as objects, the body is similarly constructed as parts of a whole. Medicine plays a large part in constructing women's bodies as parts of an object. Similarly, physicians typically discuss breast reconstruction with women who are discovering they have breast cancer in the same conversation. Ferguson argues, "By suggesting that reconstruction is a natural part of breast cancer treatment, physicians contribute to the belief that women with one or no breasts are unnatural" (Kasper and Ferguson 2000: 70). This construction of women's bodies without breasts as unnatural perpetuates an understanding of the body that is either whole or incomplete and objectified.

In contemporary culture, bodies are often represented and understood through metaphors. Susan Sontag in *Illness as Metaphor* was one of the first scholars to analyze the common tendency to discuss disease and illness through metaphor (2001). Sontag argues that cancer is often described as "invading" or "colonizing" the body (Sontag 2001: 64). Sontag (2001) argues that the military metaphor sees the body as a landscape and that metaphors of disease are a commentary about the relationship between the individual and society (Sontag 2001: 73). In "The Breast Cancer Wars" Lerner highlights the ways medicine has always used military metaphors when discussing diseases (Lerner 2000). In particular, cancer has been described with military metaphors for quite some time. Military metaphors in the context of cancer demonstrate a masculine and militarized conception of the body. According to Sontag's (2001) logic, military metaphors are also a commentary about the relationship between women and society as violent.

In *Medicine as Culture*, Deborah Lupton argues that metaphors shape our understandings of bodies with disease and as a result shape identity (Lupton 1994: 55). Lupton (1994) also assumes that bodies determine our subjectivity. Here, I would like to focus on the way metaphors construct our bodies and leave analysis of subjectivity elsewhere. Lupton (1994) highlights commonly used metaphors for the body, noting that they often include architecture, systems, or military metaphors. Lupton (1994) argues the metaphor functions to help make the body seem controllable and orderly. Lupton states, "By contrast, cancer is a disease of uncontrolled, abnormal growth that invades the body" (Lupton 1994: 58). Cancer cells are conceived of as disobedient cells. Moreover, medicine has constructed the body as something that is possible to be in control of. The body is an orderly, efficient piece of machinery that cancer disrupts.

Lupton (1994) observes that in the architectural metaphor the body is viewed as an object with clear boundaries, and parts that serve specific functions. For example, the body is conceptualized as a house and the mouth a door. In *Advanced Breast Cancer*, Musa Mayer interviewed many women to document the way women understand their own breast cancer through metaphor (Mayer 1998). Mayer states, "Jenilu Schoolman once wrote me that she had come to conceive of her body as a multi-family apartment building. Her cancer was like an unruly tenant who couldn't be evicted, but had to be kept in line and taught respect for the other inhabitants of the building" (Mayer 1998: Chapter 7). Schoolman's quote is an expression of the body constructed through architectural metaphor. Schoolman's account of her breast cancer also highlights the way the architecture metaphor locates the power within her. The ability to teach respect to the tenant is a job only Schoolman is capable of. This implies that women's breast cancer is something that may be determined by her own ability to discipline her tenant (cancer). Metaphors where women are deemed as in control can be both empowering and problematic. It is empowering for women to be in control of their bodies while facing a terrifying disease. Yet it is problematic because this creates a relationship between women and their bodies where the body should be submissive to the control of the woman's mind. It seems as though this sets a woman up for a tension-filled relationship with her body when she is unsuccessful and the cancer remains.

Lupton examines the metaphor of the "body as a computerized system" (Lupton 1994: 60). This metaphor of the body as a system maintains the body as something that can be controlled or at least programmed better. Linda Birke in "Bodies and Biology" claims we often think of health in terms of systems and maintenance (Birke 1998). As a result breast cancer adopts the rhetoric of prevention through detection. When breast cancer prevention is understood as early detection through self-exams and mammography, it becomes a maintenance of the breast as opposed to keeping the breast healthy and disease and toxic free in the first place. The breast is thought to be made of systems of fat, nodes, and ducts. The BCRA test is depicted by medical science as a technological advancement that helps determine a woman's genetic predisposition for breast cancer. In cases where the breast cancer gene is inherited, medical science views this gene as abnormal because it is not able to self-repair. In the systems metaphor, the body is viewed as parts that work together efficiently to maintain the health of the body. The breast cancer gene is unable to self-repair and therefore risks the maintenance of the system and the body. When the body is viewed as a system the implication is that women's bodies are understood as controllable. Emily Martin argues that a systems metaphor is a reflection of the hierarchical organization of contemporary society (Martin 1998: 26). According to Martin (1998), any change in the body's system is perceived as a breakdown in authority. Martin (1998) continues that cancer is feared so adamantly because it represents the breakdown of hierarchical control.

Breast cancer is discussed as invading the nodes. Similar to a computer virus cancer infects nodes systematically. We can think of cancer itself as a system gone bad. Cancer is the ultimate disruption of boundaries and systems. The systems metaphor understands the body as being controlled by systems that work efficiently. The body is commonly constructed as consisting of systems with clear boundaries. For example, the body consists of the nervous system, digestive system, and the immune system in order to name a few. Cancer disrupts the clear boundaries between bodily systems.

The call to battle against breast cancer also represents a national discourse of women as producers of better national subjects. The fight against breast cancer often rallies women by claiming this could be or has been your mother. King states:

> it becomes clear how support for the battle against the disease is frequently generated through appeals that link success in this undertaking to the preservation of national motherhood, normative femininity, and the spirit of "American generosity," even as politicians of all stripes repeatedly attest to the bipartisan and apolitical "nature" of the cause. (King 2008: 65)

In a promotional video titled "Why Walk" for the Avon Foundation, a series of reasons to walk are provided, which include "for my mom," "for my sister," "for the feeling I'm making a difference" to name a few.[18] McClintock states "nations are frequently figured through the iconography of familial and domestic space" (McClintock 1996: 262). One gentleman interviewed by the Avon Foundation, who participates in walks, states "everyone has a mother, a sister ... we never know who is going to be the next victim."[19] Breast cancer is understood here through discourses of gender in that it sees women's roles in society as their familial obligations. Notice the gentleman does not say everyone knows a CEO, a good person, or a young woman. Women are not situated by their occupation, personality, age, or other attributes they may possess as individuals in society but they are only articulated in relation to others through familial roles and specifically in relation to men.

The most common metaphor used when discussing diseased bodies is the "military metaphor" (Sontag 2001). The military metaphor positions the body as a defended territory. In this metaphor, the self is at war with the body and the weapon is Western medicine. I argue the military metaphor maintains women's bodies as a passive object to be acted upon. Lerner argues the surgeon is associated with the soldier (Lerner 2000: 70). I would argue that the surgeon is more accurately associated with a superior officer in the military providing leadership and commands. The military metaphor was embraced early on by the American Cancer Society who created the Women's Field Army (Lerner 2000: 33). This military metaphor has become more common in contemporary understandings of breast cancer.

Women fighting breast cancer are depicted as warriors. A woman who has breast cancer is said to be fighting, and battling the disease. This is not much different than other discourses of cancer but it is worth considering the way the disease is understood through metaphors of war. Moreover, in the military metaphor women's bodies are in fact the battlefields. Women's bodies in this construction are an objectified location upon which the world of medicine can act. Breast cancer has also been nationalized through metaphors of war. Metaphors of war are illustrated by Ford Motors, a major sponsor of the Susan G. Komen Foundation and the national Race for the Cure. Under the "Ford Cares" program "Calling All Warriors," individuals are asked to "Bang the drum. Paint your face. Run. Walk. Fight for the cure." It is not clear exactly what role Ford wishes to play in the breast cancer movement other than be a corporate sponsor and sell vehicles but its word choices and discourse of war are interesting and in line with common metaphors of cancer. In reality, Ford seeks participants in the National Race for the Cure after they complete their walk and passes out Ford logo items. Ford warriors can be identified through warrior gear, which includes a bandana and temporary tattoo that use pink as their primary color. This is part of Ford's campaign to promote the 2008 Mustang. In a Web site devoted to women battling inflammatory breast cancer a message states "Warrior women you join an army of wounded women, who wear pretty clothes that conceal the scars and the pain and who summon brave smiles to camouflage anxiety" (Ford 2007). The language includes bravery, camouflage, scars, and armies all of which are military phrases, terms, and sentiment. Yet it becomes difficult to understand breast cancer in any other way than the battle to live or die.

Martin argues, "Work in feminist theory suggests there is a masculinist bias to views that divide the world into sharply opposed, hostile categories, such that the options are to conquer, be conquered, or magnanimously tolerate the other" (1999: 132). Understandings of breast cancer and women's bodies that commonly employ hostile categories of conquer or be conquered reveal a masculinist bias. The military metaphor constructs the body as a violent battlefield. What is lost in a singular understanding of breast cancer as a war and the body as nation? At the very least, women with breast cancer are prevented from understanding their disease without the burden of such loaded patriarchal metaphors. Susan Sontag argues that military metaphors are dangerous because "they make people irrationally fearful of effective measures such as chemotherapy, and foster credence in thoroughly useless remedies such as diets and psychotherapy" (2001: 102). Understanding women who are in breast cancer remission as survivors is part of this war metaphor also. In conjunction with the identity of survivor, a breast cancer patient is relentlessly pressed to remain hopeful.

Lupton (2001) notes the discourse of hope surrounding cancer in general. The Avon Foundation and the Komen Foundation offer events whose primary goal is to reestablish hope in breast cancer victims and survivors. Lupton in reference to hope argues "This discourse is related to the military and invasion metaphors previously described, for it postulates that 'winning' the war against cancer is intimately linked to having a positive attitude to getting better" (Lerner 2001: 67). Breast cancer patients are asked to remain hopeful in order to combat the disease. Cancer patients are depicted as brave war heroes in this narrative (Lerner 2001: 67). In *Teratologies* Jackie Stacey (1997) argues that medicine is the hero. Stacey (1997) argues that cancer patients have the potential to become heroes if they follow the instructions of Western medicine. The military metaphor positions women as either winning the war or losing it. Since there is no cure for breast cancer, winning can only mean surviving. Survival does not ensure that the breast cancer will not return, and therefore there is no such thing as winning this war. More importantly, women's bodies understood through metaphors of war help determine medical responses toward breast cancer.

How is success measured? Since the war on breast cancer and the cause for the cure began an exorbitant amount of money has been funneled into research. There have been many positive aspects to the breast cancer health movement including increased women's awareness, more financial support for research, and screening and treatment for low-income women to name a few. However, we must ask ourselves, are our pocketbooks thinner from individual philanthropy and our conscience eased because we ran at the race for the cure? How do pink ribbons help prevent breast cancer? We should ask tough questions like are women living longer, are they getting better treatment, earlier detection, and are less women diagnosed with cancer? In 2015, the American Cancer Society estimates 1,658,370 new cases of cancer, of which 60,290 will be breast cancer, and 589,430 cancer deaths in the United States (American Cancer Society 2015). The facts are clear that prevention is necessary, and pink ribbons, consumer activism, and research for a cure are not having the necessary impact.

Notes

1. Anonymous, confidential interview by author, Boston, MA, May 2013; in author's possession.
2. Anonymous, confidential interview by author, San Francisco, CA, February 11, 2011; in author's possession.
3. Anonymous, confidential interview by author, San Francisco, CA, February 10, 2011; in author's possession.
4. Anonymous, confidential interview by author, San Rafael, CA, February 10, 2011; in author's possession.
5. Anonymous, confidential interview by author, Boston, MA, March 11, 2011; in author's possession.
6. Anonymous and confidential interview by author, Boston, MA, November 17, 2010, in author's possession.
7. Anonymous, confidential interview by author, Boston, MA, December 10, 2010; in author's possession.
8. Anonymous, confidential phone interview by author, February 28, 2011; in author's possession.
9. Anonymous, confidential interview by author, San Rafael, CA, February 10, 2011; in author's possession.
10. Anonymous, confidential interview by author, San Rafael, CA, February 10, 2011; in author's possession.
11. Anonymous, confidential interview by author, San Francisco, CA, February 10, 2011; in author's possession.
12. Anonymous, confidential interview by author, San Francisco, CA, February 10, 2011; in author's possession.
13. Anonymous, confidential interview by author, San Francisco, CA, February 8, 2011; in author's possession.
14. Anonymous, confidential phone interview by author, March 20, 2011; in author's possession.
15. Anonymous, confidential interview by author, San Francisco, CA, February 10, 2011; in author's possession.
16. Anonymous, confidential interview by author, San Francisco, CA, February 8, 2011; in author's possession.
17. Anonymous, confidential phone interview by author, February 28, 2011; in author's possession.
18. Avon Foundation, "Why Walk," http://walk.avonfoundation.org, May 16, 2007.
19. Avon Foundation, "Avon Walk Videos," http://walk.avon foundation.org , May 16, 2007.

CHAPTER 5

Conclusion

At the 2011 National Breast Cancer Coalition (NBCC) conference, Dr. Susan Love, founder of the Army of Women, issued a call for women to use not only their contributions but also their voices and bodies to improve medical research and stop breast cancer:

> Medical researchers say women are too messy and we can't control them and this is why they use mice and rats. Yet we need research on women if we are going to figure this out. It is time that we now say it was one thing to wear pink and raise money and that is all good, but if we want to stop breast cancer, then we have to have a plan. The NBCC has always been at the forefront of this. If we launch and push forward and demand and yell and scream and join the Army of Women, we can't tell them we want more research and then have no women who will be a part of it.[1]

Dr. Love clearly sees women in a position of power and as central to stopping breast cancer. In March 2011, the Army of Women sent an e-mail in honor of Women's History Month that listed key women's rights pioneers and their accomplishments and stated, "We have the power as women, as mothers, daughters, sisters and friends to make breast cancer a part of our history. Together, women have changed history before and the Army of Women is on a mission to do it again" (Army of Women 2011). Dr. Love and the Army of Women thus remind us of the embodied nature of breast cancer and the power of women to advocate change. This chapter explores the connections between the breast cancer movement and other social movements such as women's rights. Green organizations like Breast Cancer Fund (BCF) and Breast Cancer Action (BCA) have been very successful at partnering with like-minded organizations outside of the breast cancer movement, yet pink organizations have not yet made some of these connections. Connections to other social movements like the motherhood movement, women's rights, environment, and AIDS are opportunities that may help fulfill the promise of prevention. Building coalitions and networks across social movements represents a future direction for breast cancer advocacy and one way that the promise of prevention might be fulfilled.

Social Movements Spillover and Intramovement Dynamics

The breast cancer movement exists in relation to other social movements such as the women's health movement, the AIDS activist health movement, and the environmental health movement (Turshen 2007). By understanding the breast cancer movement and advocacy organizations, as connected to and informed by other social movements, we can move beyond individual case studies and explore how health-based social movements function (Brown and Zavestoski 2005). Brown and Zavestoski (2005) using Meyer and Whittier (1994) understand this relationship as "social movement spillover" (Brown and Zavestoski 2005: 8). In other words the women's health movement, AIDS movement, and environmental health movement have affected the shape of the breast cancer movement.

"Social movement spillover" is particularly evident in the breast cancer advocacy groups with a greener agenda during the 1990s. Ulrike Boehmer's (2000) *The Personal and the Political* argued many breast cancer organizations have a history of working with, and being influenced by, earlier social movements such as civil rights and AIDS activism. Many of the advocates I interviewed cited the AIDS movement and its challenge to federal research as the inspiration that mobilized them to found key organizations like BCA. Specifically, BCA cites the AIDS movement as quite influential in BCA's early days of advocacy. Brendtro argued, "Breast Cancer activists took their cues from AIDS activists in identifying successful strategies to bring breast cancer to the national health care agenda" (1998: 3). Both movements sought to end shame around the disease as well as increase funding for research. Turshen (2007) argues that ACT UP, founded in 1987, is an example of a grassroots community response to the AIDS epidemic that demanded that more research and treatment options be made available (Turshen 2007: 88). In addition members of the AIDS activist movement were actively challenging medical research and pushing for more government funding, which organizations like BCA and BCF pursue in their strategic actions (Brown et al. 2004). Klawiter (2008) stated BCA learned a great deal from AIDS activist organizations; she states "From ACT UP they learned how to make sense of articles in medical journals, how to work with media, how to apply pressure to pharmaceutical companies and government agencies, and how to chain themselves to the fence if all else failed" (Klawiter 2008: 173). The AIDS activist organizations used confrontational and often disruptive strategies to gain attention and support for their cause. Boehmer, in *The Personal and the Political*, asks why women get involved with the HIV/AIDS movement versus the breast cancer movement. Boehmer conducted 37 interviews with individuals who are members of organizations, participated in activism, or were paid workers in breast cancer and AIDS organizations for an average of five years. The author finds that women participate because of interpersonal ties and relationships and/or a political tie and interest in feminist or women's activism. In other words, some individuals participate because the disease personally affects them, while others participate because they are already activists around women's issues or health issues. For example, some activists are involved in breast cancer activism because they are already involved in feminist organizations like the National Organization for Women (NOW) or they are involved in AIDS activism. Boehmer found that women who engage in breast cancer activism tend to understand social disadvantage only in the terms of gender inequality. In other words, women who are breast cancer activists focus solely on a gendered inequality of how the disease affects women. Women who choose HIV/AIDS activism think of social inequities in terms of racial, class, gender, and sexuality. Boehmer found that those who participate in HIV/AIDS activism have a tendency toward an understanding of race, class, and gender as intersecting to form inequality. While Boehmer's main investigation was into mobilization of advocates she does not see organizations' principled beliefs and strategies as playing a crucial role. Instead her conclusions help us to understand why similar health-based movements differ.

Presently, there are some connections being made to the U.S. motherhood movement, environmental health, and breast cancer groups. Interestingly, several respondents cited a link between the environmental movement, breast cancer movement, and motherhood movement as very common and powerful. For example, MomsRising is an organization that several respondents cited being affiliated with.

MomsRising is an online network that focuses on maternity leave, employment issues for mothers, breast-feeding politics, and toxins in beauty products and food. MomsRising came up in several of the interviews at BCF specifically. A member of the board of directors at BCF articulates the link between the motherhood movement, environmental health, and breast cancer advocacy:

> Young mothers get very outraged when they learn about the oversights of the government and MomsRising (started by Moveon.org) speaks to that. We honored MomsRising in helping pass legislation to ban toxins in toys. The members mobilized and called and wrote letters and they were an important part of what we do which is education and reaction.[2]

The BCF's work with MomsRising represents an interesting coalition between environmental health advocacy and the motherhood movement. A staff member and activist who works on Bisphenol A (BPA) with the Safe Cosmetics Alliance reflected on why the environmental health movement mobilizes women: "The environmental health movement has more women. Women are more in tune with their bodies and pay attention to new movements. They are more conscious. It grabs women as mothers."[3] Certainly the environmental justice movement in the United States has been largely populated by women of color and mothers (Stein 2004). In the case of MomsRising and the overlap to breast cancer, the identity of motherhood as a location for advocacy seems significant. The interviewees suggest that women are more likely to be involved in environmental health advocacy because they are mothers out of concern for their children's health and well-being. MomsRising is articulating messages that overlap with the BCF with regard to BPA and toxins in our personal care, cleaning products, food, and toys.

Breast Cancer as a Women's Rights Issue

Although several organizations expressed the desire to network and work with "women's rights" organizations, few saw this as a "women's" issue or as "women's rights" or even a "women's health issue." For example, a staff member at BCA responded to a question about whether activism is connected to other social movements and specifically the women's movement by saying,

When you look at it as a woman's rights issue, you get pissed off. When perhaps she has a disease that may kill her based on environmental exposure. I know a number of women that don't want to get pissed off. They have the disease, they have gone through the mastectomy, and they just want to get on with their lives. I don't think women are encouraged to be rowdy and unruly.[4]

Her words demonstrate the importance of interrogating the way traditional gender expectations of women as passive, cooperative, nice, and soft play into a lack of connection between women's rights and breast cancer advocacy. However, her comments direct our attention to a key insight that many women are just trying to survive and live and advocacy for breast cancer prevention or women's rights is not a priority. Survival is the priority. Yet it seems there are missed connections between breast cancer advocacy and the women's movements, which merit further research because the participants in this study cited examples where this could be a beneficial partnership.

Only one organization, the BCA, self-identified as feminist, although the BCF does cite coalitions to women's rights organizations like Sistersong, which is a feminist reproductive justice organization. Most organizations saw breast cancer activism as part of a larger health-based activism or part of a larger environmental movement rather than a feminist issue or a women's rights issue. One participant, a former CEO of the Komen Foundation, argued that women have been empowered by the breast cancer movement because it has given a credible voice to women and their doctors and politicians that did not exist before.[5] In other words, the breast cancer movement has opened up opportunities for women's empowerment, voice, and political action. Similarly, one staff member from BCF articulates the view that the breast cancer advocacy work on toxins in our products is closely aligned with a women's health movement, understanding that women have the right to control their bodies. She states:

I think that *Our Bodies Our Selves* model of women's right to have authority over their bodies, what enters it and what leaves it, even reproductive rights, people have the right to make decisions about when they want to have children. They also have the right to have a healthy child if they want to have a child. I think there are bridges with any number of components with the women's health and women's rights in overt ways.[6]

A staff member who works for the Campaign for Safe Cosmetics (which is in coalition with the BCF) argues that breast cancer organizations are more closely aligned with environmental organizations rather than women's rights organizations. However, she sees that more connections are being made to women's organizations like Planned Parenthood:

> The prevention organizations started to align more with environmental justice and they have a ways to go. I think they are aware of that and I hope that with funding, and with clear priorities that will happen. With reproductive health groups and women's rights groups, this is becoming much more of a salient connection. Just in the past couple of years, I worked with Planned Parenthood with their green choices initiative and really helped to frame some of the messaging around why we must be aware of toxic chemicals and how they are impacting fertility.[7]

In this case of Planned Parenthood there is an understanding that toxic chemicals impact fertility not just cancer risk. This demonstrates an understanding of prevention that has been advocated by green organizations. Even though most advocacy organizations did not express the connection between breast cancer and women's rights, if we examine the NOW as just one example of a women's rights organization, we see breast health as important to women's rights. The NOW does consider breast cancer a woman's health and rights issue.

In 1999, NOW's president Patricia Ireland temporarily joined forces with the BCF and members of Congress to ask for funding for research into the causes of breast cancer and specifically environmental factors. The NOW's statement makes three demands: increased funding, access to screening and care regardless of income or age, and research on environmental links. According to the NOW,

> Environmentalists and feminists alike share a common interest in research on the effect of environmental degradation on women's health. This concern is reflected in the many women's rights activists who identify themselves as eco-feminists and the many environmental activists who are strong women's rights supporters. Now, we must challenge the scientific research community and policy makers to look for answers to the questions that plague every woman who has ever felt a lump in her breast: Why does this

happen? How can we prevent it? And how can we cure it? (Ireland 1999)

In 2000, the NOW began to build coalitions with members of Congress and 70 organizations working on breast cancer causes in order to understand the environmental risk factors. The BCF specifically worked with Patricia Ireland and Representative Nancy Pelosi (D-CA) to ask publicly for support of this women's health issue and to look for prevention. The NOW also demands that more research be done regarding the risk of breast implants with regard to cancer (NOW 2000).

In 2004, NOW released a statement "Pink Ribbons Everywhere," supporting events like the BCA's "Think before You Pink" campaign that encourages women to be critical of pink cause–related marketing. The NOW points out that some cosmetic companies who raise money for cancer also sell products that contain chemicals linked to cancer. Similarly in 2010, the NOW's blog for equality posted an article criticizing Facebook campaigns asking women to post their bra color on their wall in support of breast cancer awareness. The NOW criticizes such a campaign as exploiting women's bodies and ignoring any meaningful call to action against breast cancer (Karbon 2010). In this regard the NOW is taking on a prevention-based message and a critical perspective of pink ribbons, which is a perspective found primarily in green breast cancer organizations.

Susan G. Komen does use a women's empowerment message as evident in some of its brochures. Although it does not make any formal connections to women's rights organizations to fight breast cancer, it does provide funding for breast health and early detection to Planned Parenthood, arguably a women's rights organization. While Komen has not built coalitions with women's rights groups, it uses a discourse of women's empowerment to advocate breast health. The Susan G. Komen for the Cure's 2007 brochure gives us an insight into the ideational links between women's rights, equality, and the breast cancer movement. The brochure (notably all pink) stated, "We're looking for some women to work around the house" (Komen Foundation 2007). Upon opening the brochure, a photo of the White House is featured, yet it is not asking for increased political representation. Instead what it is asking for is women advocates to lobby their representatives. Susan G. Komen's purposeful use of equality rhetoric is evident when it states "Breast Cancer is an equal-opportunity disease. So are our efforts" (2007). Other examples of discourse of female empowerment include a 2010 pink promise ring for the cure stated, "Empower Yourself with Knowledge." Each of these examples shows that pink organizations like Komen do see the connections to women's rights and empowerment but are not using them as an organizational strategy in the ways that green breast cancer organizations are.

Breast cancer advocacy has been influenced by environmental justice activism, women's rights, women's health, and AIDS activism, making clear that there has been social movement spillover. Moreover, the breast cancer movement, as evidenced by green organizations coalitions and networks, seeks to make these social movement connections more formal. More importantly, the coalitions and intra-movement advocacy networks continue to evolve and grow in importance. The results from this research indicate the growing importance of networks and coalitions to advocacy organizations who operate as niche-based organizations.

Diversity

Scholars like Boehmer (2000) have noted the lack of racial/ethnic, gender, class, and age diversity within the breast cancer movement. The demographic data collected for this study demonstrate that gender, race, and age are overwhelmingly similar within and across the organizations examined. The majority of individuals working at the breast cancer organizations examined in this study were highly educated white women. Almost all participants in the study discussed the lack of racial and class diversity within the movement, and expressed their concerns. In terms of age, many organizations were proud of their ability to get younger women involved, yet the majority of interviewees felt that the organizations and the movement needed a lot more diversity. Andrews and Edwards (2004) argued that the literature on advocacy organizations and membership has shown that privileged persons are more likely to respond to recruitment. In this way the breast cancer advocate demographic is not surprising. For example, in the case of breast cancer advocacy, those with economic privilege have the time and resources to mobilize and participate in breast cancer advocacy. Strolovich (2007) argued that advocacy organizations pursue strategies and policies that reflect the majority of their membership, and therefore, if the majority of an organization's membership and staff is made up of middle- and upper-class white women, an organization will pursue policies and campaigns that affect that group. Boehmer supports this finding; she states "Generally it can be stated that cancer activism is now shaped from the racial perspective of whiteness and a middle-class background. This means that concerns of non-white communities and poor women are mostly excluded" (2000: 122).

Nonetheless, Strolovich argued, "concerns about representing disadvantaged subgroups weigh heavily on the minds of organization officers, and the majority of them are genuinely committed to the goal of advocacy for their multiply disadvantaged constituents" (2007: 8). Similarly, this study's findings show that there is a stated commitment to representing disadvantaged groups and increasing diversity within the organization, although this does not always translate into strategies and policies to ensure diversity nor does it increase diversity in terms of membership, staff, or board of directors' participation. For example, the Army of Women is in the process of conducting focus groups of women of color to see if the Army of Women message is getting across and to better understand why there are so few women of color in its database. Some organizations acknowledged that they needed to be more diverse, but were unclear how to achieve this other than networking through coalitions. These organizations did not seem to have a clear organizational strategy for increasing diversity. For example, the Breast Cancer Coalition (BCC) in San Francisco, which receives grant money from Komen, provides materials in roughly a dozen languages but stated it is uncertain how to get non-English-speaking women into its office and involved in its work. In the case of San Francisco BCC the desire to expand membership across race, class, and gender demographics existed but the necessary strategies to do so were unclear.

In addition, a few people I interviewed from the Komen Foundation felt that this issue of diversity was changing, in part due to a commitment by Komen to draw in diverse groups through grants and community-level events and educational sessions. For example, the Susan G. Komen for the Cure has developed a "Circle of Promise," a pledge to

> ensure that African American women are empowered with the information and tools they need to take charge of their own health and serve as ambassadors in their local communities. The Circle of Promise movement is designed to engage African American women to help end breast cancer forever by fostering increased awareness, support, empowerment and action. (Komen Foundation 2010)

Susan G. Komen was the exception in that it had implemented specific strategies to increase diversity within the movement and its membership base. Moreover, a staff member from the Boston Komen chapter stated,

> At the very beginning when you look at Komen, Komen is seen as a very affluent white women's organization. Here at the local level we are changing that perception. We are really engaging all individual racial and ethnic populations from Portuguese, Cape Verdean, Brazilian, Asian American population I think that is something as an organization we really want to go ahead and continue cultivating relationships in those communities. I think we have been able to tap in every racial and ethnic community to ensure that we are as a brand very powerful. Within an organization we have a conscious effort since I have been on board to ensure that we are the face of all women and their families of the commonwealth and not only the white affluent women.[8]

Clearly, Susan G. Komen has shown that it is committed to diversity in more than principle and has actively engaged in programs and campaigns designed to be inclusive. According to a Komen participant,

> It starts from the grant making process to ensure that we have a really diverse portfolio of organizations that we are funding. And that reaching certain segments of the population, are very diverse. And when I mean diversity I don't only mean racial and ethnic, I mean regionally that this is a statewide organization and that women in the West cannot be forgotten especially if you look at funding streams around the state of Massachusetts, there are so many organizations funded here in the city of Boston. We want to ensure that we are spread out throughout the commonwealth. I look at the economic piece that is really important to have an understanding of the economic realities of so many women in the commonwealth and the financial hardship they face during treatment.[9]

In the case of Susan G. Komen there is an effort to expand notions of diversity beyond race, class, and gender to a more inclusive regional impact. In other words, Susan G. Komen wanted to ensure its local chapters were reaching all areas of the state, not just urban areas. This represents an important point as most breast cancer advocacy groups are located in urban areas.

A program associate at BCA states,

> breast cancer is the leading cancer among Latinas, and while they have a lower incidence than Caucasian women have, it is rising for Latina's. That is something we are trying to do and meeting with Latina leaders and trying to inform women about breast cancer and reducing risk … I feel as if the larger breast cancer movement has had the unfortunate problem of speaking to primarily financially privileged white women who are educated—and that obscures the fact that breast cancer is largely an environmental disease. It is low-income communities of color who are disproportionately affected by exposure to unhealthy environments and who typically have greater risk of mortality from breast cancer. There's environmental exposure and then there is also the issue of healthcare access and I feel as if the larger movement has glossed over that.[10]

Although breast cancer does affect women of all races and classes, it affects women of different race and class backgrounds in unique ways. For example, according to the National Cancer Institute, African American women have a lower survival rate than white women (National Cancer Institute 2010). In advocacy by Susan G. Komen, the rhetoric is that breast cancer could affect all women regardless of race, age, and class (Braun 2003). She is articulating an important point that breast cancer is an issue relevant to all women but fails to draw our attention to the way that breast cancer affects women of color and working class women in particularly detrimental ways. Braun argued that it is possible for all women to get breast cancer, but does not articulate the way social inequality affects the health and life of a person with cancer.

The argument by Braun (2003) is representative of mainstream breast cancer activism and it leads us to believe that race, class, and age are less significant for this women's health issue, when in fact the opposite is true. Brown (2007) articulates the point that inequality correlates to worse health and increased risk of breast cancer. Yet, when mainstream breast cancer activism emphasizes the universality of women's experience of breast cancer; this marginalizes the reality that breast cancer is not the same for all women (Avon Foundation 2007; Komen Foundation 2010). Yet we do see a more recent effort by Susan G. Komen, Avon, and NBCC to highlight the role racial inequalities play on one's health. For example, Susan G. Komen's "Circle of Promise

Campaign for African American Women" and its advisory councils for particular populations such as Hispanic and Latina, African American, Asian American, and American Indian women demonstrate an effort to formally consider ways to address racial diversity (Komen Foundation 2010). The environmentally based breast cancer movement seems to begin with the premise that race and class do affect a women's experience with breast cancer and the types of activism she will engage in.

Advocacy versus Activism: I'm Not an Activist But . . .

The responses to the initial requests for informants to participate in this research project revealed an interesting finding: participants in the breast cancer movement do not identify themselves as "activists" but prefer to identify as "advocates." I found that the word *activist* was a contentious term at worst and a meaningless term at best among participants within the breast cancer movement. After a few organizations agreed to post my call for research participants in their newsletter, several women contacted me stating they would like to be involved but were not sure if they were suitable, as they did not consider themselves activists, the term used in my initial request. Two women even wrote me e-mails challenging my use of the term and suggesting that I cease using the word activist, stating adamantly that women fighting against breast cancer were advocates.[11] Because the term *advocate* was what most respondents appeared to identify with, and the qualitative interviews supported a definition of advocacy, I believe that the breast cancer organizations and the individual participants in this book are best understood as advocacy organizations and as health-based advocates. Earp, French, and Gilkey's (2007) *Patient Advocacy for Health Care Quality* distinguishes between three types of patient advocacy. The first type of advocacy includes the work done by "helping professions" such as nurses and social work, the second type includes care-specific advocacy that focuses on patient autonomy such as palliative care, and the third type is activists connected to social movements (2007: 6–8). In other words, they argue that activism is a type of advocacy where the aim is to improve healthcare for marginalized groups. Defining advocacy is an important step as the literatures of nonprofit, advocacy, and social movements overlap. Advocates seek to influence their communities and sometimes policies. Prakash and Gugerty stated,

> The term "advocacy" suggests systematic efforts (as opposed to sporadic outbursts) by actors that seek to further specific policy

goals. Advocacy is integral to politics and not restricted to any particular policy domain. It could pertain to environmental protection, labor issues, healthcare issues, religion, democracy, shareholders' rights and so on. (2010: 1)

Breast cancer advocates have a vision of how things should be in terms of breast cancer services, care, and research and they set about to make that vision happen through policy change and ideational campaigns aimed at changing understandings of cancer. However advocacy is more than "seeking to further specific policy goals" (Prakash and Gugerty 2010: 1). A commonly cited definition by Jenkins (1987) is "any attempt to influence the decisions of an institutional elite on behalf of a collective interest" (Jenkins 1987: 297). Jenkins's (1987) definition of advocacy is quite inclusive and would cover organizational activities beyond influencing policy. Breast cancer organizations do much more than attempt to shape policy, such as translating scientific findings, reframing understandings of disease and medical research, and increasing awareness about this disease. In this case, advocates aim to influence institutional elites such as policy makers, scientists, and medical researchers on behalf of the collective interests of women.

Activism and advocacy are quite similar in that they both involve making claims on behalf of a collective group to achieve social change. However, activism is political in nature and often involves protest tactics whereas advocacy does not necessarily have to be explicitly political or involve protest tactics. Is there, ironically, a political reason then that advocates refuse the label activists? They do not want to alienate potential donors with any kind of formal political affiliations. The 1990s' green breast cancer organizations would best be understood as activist in large part because of their use of protest tactics like toxic tours, die-ins, and picketing walks for the cure. Today, however, both pink and green movements no longer utilize activist tactics as they did in the 1990s. Instead they make collective interest claims by trying to shape policy, educate the public, and shape the research agenda. Therefore, after the initial pilot interviews, I changed the language in the call for participants' letter to *advocate*, which elicited more willingness and interest from women to participate in the research. This less overtly political approach also supports the definition of advocacy provided by Andrews and Edwards (2004), which understands advocates as those who make public interest claims to achieve social change and focus on policy and education.

A policy coordinator at BCF states,

> I consider myself probably more of an advocate than an activist. I come from activist roots. I got into the world of public policy through the National Organization for Women, which was absolutely activism and sort of on the streets, vigils, and marches, and all that stuff. I don't do a lot of that direction action stuff now. But I definitely consider myself an advocate and somebody who seeks to change the world by convincing people the worthiness of the cause.[12]

Nonetheless, in the process of doing the qualitative interviews, some women, after defining the term *activist* for themselves, decided they were in fact activists. For example, a volunteer for Susan Love's Army of Women (sponsored by the Avon Foundation), and a member and participant in Avon foundation events, thoughtfully considered whether she might be an activist:

> An *activist* is not the word I would use. However, when I was talking with my boyfriend and read him your questions, he disagreed. He said that I am an activist because I am putting all of my energy into this and every opportunity I have, I am thinking about breast cancer and what more I can do. So yes, I do fit that definition of an activist. However, the word *activist* has a very negative connotation as though you are burning down buildings to get attention. The pink energy and noise is too positive to be activism. I think of activists as antiwar or green peace and so I haven't associated that word with what I am doing.[13]

It is interesting that she was willing to reframe her own work to fight breast cancer as activism. It is clear that "activist" has come to have a negative connotation for many people, but it seems especially so in this case because pink and the specific strategies Avon uses, such as physical walks like "In It to End It," have an upbeat, hopeful, and positive message that finding a cure is possible, implying that activism is downbeat and negative, confined to burning down buildings.

After completing the interviews, a clear exception to the a negative association of *activist* with an angry trouble-maker holding a picket sign were the interviews with participants from the BCA and BCF in San Francisco. For example, when asked whether she was an activist and what that means, one participant stated, "It means not sitting by. Signing petitions, boycotting, a certain store, talking about certain issues to friends, somewhat posting on Facebook. . . . The actions have a collective impact."[14]

Despite political disavowals, the language used by the Susan G. Komen Foundation is that of activism. For example, one brochure states, "Through Komen Champions for the Cure, we use the power of activism to achieve important legislative objectives at federal, state, and local levels" (Komen Foundation 2007: 1). Komen frequently refers to itself as a network of survivors and activists. A staff member at the Boston chapter of Susan G. Komen offered this definition: "Activism means really engaging community and cultivating key partnerships with stakeholders at the local level to really move an agenda forward."[15] Despite the objections of many of the research participants in this book, Susan G. Komen is nonetheless one of the most widely known breast cancer organization and mobilizes people in record numbers, suggesting that its use of the language of activism has not raised any significant objections or prevented mobilization. Komen's Advocacy Alliance has focused on policy such as the Affordable Care Act and encouraged increased funding of breast cancer research. It stated,

> The Susan G. Komen for the Cure® Advocacy Alliance takes a stand on issues of importance to cancer survivors, advocates, and others involved in the movement. Primarily, our positions relate to breast cancer research, early detection, and access to high-quality care. From time to time, we may also comment on other health-related topics and sign onto letters published by other organizations, which we feel may have an impact on the breast cancer community. (Komen Foundation 2012)

Notably Komen's advocacy work is a smaller component than other large-scale organizations like NBCC for which advocacy is a primary goal rather than a secondary one. Here we see Susan G. Komen create a branch within its organization devoted to advocacy while the majority of the work Susan G. Komen does uses the language of activism. By identifying themselves as advocates, participants made clear in the interviews that they advocated for policy change (so do activists) on the basis of research for the cure or prevention and environmental health concerns.

Networks and Coalitions among Organizations and Activists

Breast cancer organizations have focused a great deal on fund-raising, but they also try to raise awareness and influence policy through the use of coalitions and networks. This book adds to the literature on advocacy organizations precisely because it attempts to better understand the intraorganizational differences and dynamics that make up the larger field of the breast cancer movement. A network is a relation linking persons, objects, or events (Knoke and Yang 2008; Mitchell 1969). Networks are measured by examining linkages to other social movements, activists, and organizations as identified in interviews and surveys. Heaney and McClurg support this approach and argue that network analysis is conducive to many types of methods, including surveys and interviews, despite the fact that networks are often measured quantitatively (2009: 729). The larger breast cancer movement networks and coalitions are increasingly being used as a key strategy.

In the previous chapters, it was argued that advocacy organizations seek to carve out a niche for themselves within their issue domain. It is useful to consider how breast cancer advocacy organizations see themselves in relation to each other and perceive the role they play in the larger movement. Many of the organizations researched perceived themselves in isolation or as a "lone wolf" in their specific niche or area of expertise. For example, the Zero Breast Cancer, BCF, and NBCC all expressed the view that there were very few voices in the breast cancer movement articulating the view that the environment is linked to cancer. This implies that advocacy organizations on some level see themselves as unique and somewhat isolated from other breast cancer advocacy organizations.

Alternatively, we also see many advocacy organizations building coalitions and networks with other like-minded breast cancer organizations. Prakash and Gugerty stated,

If they cannot effectively pursue a policy goal alone, they might create or join networks or alliances and pool resources with like-minded NGOs. Even when working in networks with like-minded actors, however, NGO activists are unlikely to be oblivious to the imperatives of organizational survival. As in the case of firms, cooperation and competition will go hand in hand. NGOs will seek to protect their interests, especially to take credit if their efforts succeed; after all, publicity is the oxygen for advocacy organizational survival. (2010: 11)

In the breast cancer movement while many organizations may perceive themselves as a "lone wolf," they also see the importance of working together on key issues.

The case of the Susan G. Komen for the Cure is the clearest example of the influence of networks. In the Komen Foundation the founder Nancy Brinker's individual political networks and more importantly the level of influence, power, and wealth she has networked into played a substantial role in the early success of the Komen Foundation. Presently, the Susan G. Komen for the Cure seeks to cultivate relationships with like-minded organizations primarily through their grantees according to a participant from Komen. The Susan G. Komen for the Cure saw its grantee program as a key organizational strategy to reach new members, create change in the local community, and increase organizational diversity. The networking with other organizations through the grantee program was an institutionalized networking where Komen benefits from association with organizations that emphasize screening, access, and awareness. Moreover, smaller breast cancer organizations benefit from the level of funding and resources Susan G. Komen has access to. In this sense, it is a mutually beneficial network or smaller local-level breast cancer organizations.

In 1982, the National Alliance of Breast Cancer Organizations (NABCO), best characterized as a pink organization (King 2008: xv), was formed to distribute necessary information for women living with breast cancer. NABCO serves as an early example of the relationship between breast cancer organization, corporations, and politics. As King (2008) pointed out, most of NABCO's funding came from pharmaceutical companies (xv). NABCO did not attempt to challenge the federal research agenda but rather distributed information for women and has been criticized by many scholars and advocates as showing the early problematic partnerships between corporations that profit from cancer and a movement seeking to end cancer. (NABCO disbanded in 2004, as the movement became saturated with advocacy organizations with similar focus.) Although NABCO provides a key example of efforts to formally connect breast cancer organizations and advocates, it also fostered corporate and political relationships as well and did not make efforts to challenge the research agenda or to shape public policy but served more as an information-based organization where women could get up-to-date information on cancer or where women in treatment could buy such products as wigs (King 2008: xv). In particular, this key breast cancer organization did not challenge the federal research agenda as other health-based social movements such as the AIDS movement were at the time (King 2008: xv).

One of the most interesting things is the relationship between smaller organizations such as Silent Spring Institute (this is the Massachusetts-based environmental research group investigating Cape Cod cancer incidence) and the national-level organizations like the Avon Foundation. Although the Silent Spring Institute was founded in part by the Massachusetts Breast Cancer Coalition (MBCC), and its focus is on environmental links to cancer, its funding is quite interesting. The Silent Spring is partially funded by Avon, as are several of the smaller environmentally based organizations in California and Massachusetts. Silent Spring receives millions of dollars from the Avon Foundation for example. In other words, these organizations are connected through funding even if they may not be in a formal coalition or network.

As it turns out, the world of breast cancer advocacy is highly connected. In *Mobilizing Science*, McCormick (2009) demonstrates the many connections between breast cancer organizations in the San Francisco, Massachusetts, and Long Island areas on a national level and local level. McCormick argued that there are connections between the NBCC, BCF, BCA, MBCC, and Silent Spring, among others (see McCormick 2009: Figure 1.1 EBCM Movement Organizational Chart). Instead of viewing the world of breast cancer advocacy in isolation, it is more useful to view it as highly interconnected. Many advocates belong to multiple breast cancer organizations simultaneously. Staff and board members are often involved with multiple advocacy organizations precisely because each organization has something unique to offer them. Moreover, breast cancer advocacy organizations often work together on key issues or campaigns. Each breast cancer organization stated it wished there was more networking and collaboration among breast cancer groups. The majority used the terms "niche" to describe their work. For some groups, this was an intentional strategy to differentiate themselves from other breast cancer groups as discussed in Chapter 2. Yet, they all stated they wished to work together more and desire networks and formal connections.

Networks and coalitions are a key strategy of the smaller breast cancer organizations. When an organization wishes to get involved in a particular issue but perceives that they do not have the resources or capabilities, they will form coalitions. Barakso (2010) argued that an organization's tactical focus is an important factor in whether coalitions will be used. For example, the BCF has built partnerships with the Safe Cosmetics Campaign and the Safer Chemicals organization. Two participants who both worked on the Safe Cosmetics Campaign expressed their perception that working on the links between carcinogens in products and cancer was very important but as an organization could not take on such a big issue so they partner with different organizations in the form of coalitions. The main reason to build coalitions is to align the health-based constituency of environmental justice, environmental health, and breast cancer groups. In this way, there is support for common causes.

The Way Forward

This book has provided a comparative analysis of pink and green breast cancer advocacy organizations by assessing organizational policies, characteristics, internal structure, model programs, tactics, advocacies, and inclusiveness within breast cancer organizations. The findings of this study answer three research questions:

1. How do pink and green breast cancer organizations differ in terms of organizational policies, characteristics, internal structure, model programs, tactics, advocacies, and diversity?
2. How do these factors explain why breast cancer organizations prefer green or pink activism?
3. Are the goals of pink and green organizations converging or diverging?

I have shown that the pink and green aspects of breast cancer advocacy have converged toward a greener focus within the breast cancer movement. Moreover, I have argued that individual organizations have operated to capture a specific niche and as the mission of the larger movement converges, organizations will have to adapt and modify their niche. This study draws from social movement, breast cancer, and feminist literature to offer an innovative look at advocacy groups who participate in two principal forms of breast cancer activism: "pink" or mainstream activism and "green" or environmental activism. The results contribute to three sets of scholarly literature: social science research (from political science and sociology) on social movements and advocacy organizations, particularly that which examines the importance of social networks; social science research on breast cancer activism, much of which could be understood as a subset of the social movement field; and the still broader area of feminist theory.

This study also contributes to the current literature on advocacy organizations, supporting Andrews and Edwards's argument that the current literature on advocacy organizations can be enhanced by stronger qualitative research on organizations and issue domains, focusing on small and local advocacy organizations on a specific health issue, and pursuing a qualitative research design (2000: 500). In addition, by examining both large national advocacy organizations and small local advocacy organizations, this book contributes to the literature on organizations.

Lastly, this book contributes to the breast cancer literature by adopting the original perspective that advocacy groups are best understood as converging on the issue of prevention, which stands in contrast to previous scholarship on submovements within a larger movement. It is also one of the few studies in this literature that specifically looks at organizations themselves systematically and in depth, putting advocacy organizations rather than individuals at the forefront of its analysis. In Chapter 1 I argued that the breast cancer movement is an embodied health movement and that the larger movement is undergoing a paradigm shift toward environmental connections to cancer. Chapter 2 has provided a history and description of the types of advocacy organizations found in the movement. Its historical narrative of the breast cancer movement demonstrates that there is no longer a clear pink and green divide between advocacy organizations. I have argued that understandings of prevention, coupled with the desire of advocacy organizations to create a niche, demonstrate a greening of the larger movement. Moreover, this book contributes to the existing literature by offering a qualitative research study that demonstrates the ways advocacy organizations often behave like firms in a policy market (e.g., Prakash and Gugerty 2010) and build a specific niche and brand identity for themselves (e.g., Barakso 2010). The various understandings of prevention found in both pink and green demonstrate the nature of the shift in the larger movement. Chapter 3 has uncovered a wider pattern in the breast cancer movement through an examination of advocacy organization's strategies. This pattern is the adoption of strategies to create scientific knowledge, build expertise, and disseminate scientific information. This chapter finds that Web-based strategies are a key aspect of advocacy organization's actions and concludes that material resources play a key role in shaping an organization's strategy to fight for prevention. Chapter 4 takes on the pink ribbon and consumer activism. I examined organizations' stance on corporate donations and partnerships and pink ribbon products. Chapter 5 has explored the social movement spillover and coalitions across social movements and future directions for research on breast cancer advocacy including women's rights coalitions, diversity, and defining activism. I have shown that the breast cancer movement is shifting away from what I call the pink toward a green environmental approach to cancer, and I argued the contentious nature of pink ribbons and the consumer-based activism it. I have demonstrated the importance of citizen–science alliances to the breast cancer movements and their aims to democratize science. In conclusion, breast cancer advocacy not only demands access to health care, but also utilizes the embodied experiences of individuals as a way of pursuing its strategies.

Breast cancer was once thought to affect privileged white women in America. Now it has become clear that breast cancer is a disease that affects women regardless of nationality, race, or global position. According to the World Health Organization (WHO), cancer in general is the leading cause of death around the world causing 7.6 million deaths in the year 2005 (World Health Organization 2008a). The WHO reports that specifically breast cancer causes 502,000 deaths per year (World Health Organization 2008a). Of all cancer deaths world wide, 70% occur in low- and middle-income countries because of lack of resources (World Health Organization 2008a). This demonstrates that the mortality rate, level of treatment, and prevention are greatly dependent on nationality and class. Breast cancer is clearly a disease that women across the globe face and more and more women are seeking ways to fight this disease across national boundaries. Breast cancer activism consists of purchase pink campaigns, races for the cure, and other fitness-based events; fund-raising for scientific research; and support groups for women with breast cancer. These have been the traditional modes of breast cancer activism being utilized by breast cancer activist organizations.

As a result U.S.-based breast cancer organizations like the Komen and Avon foundations are going transnational. In September of 2007, the Komen Foundation held an international conference in Budapest, demonstrating a commitment to transnational feminist activism. The problematic relationships between consumer activism, corporate sponsorship, and women's bodies become an even greater problem as the Avon and Komen foundations are actively trying to "go global." The Avon Foundation through the "Walk around the World" tries to establish women are linked through their common fight against breast cancer (Avon Foundation 2008). It has implemented a

"Global Connection Ribbon Ceremony" where women pass the pink ribbon to survivors across the globe. The exportation of the pink ribbon may have different cultural meanings around the world. Hopefully it will not signify a rigid notion of women's femininity but rather could become a more productive symbol. Interestingly the ribbon itself has been renamed as the global connection ribbon. Perhaps this is because the color pink does not have the same symbolic impact in other countries as it does in the United States. The Avon Foundation's global fight against breast cancer does assume women share common problems across the globe and this is potentially problematic given feminist theories' critique against global feminism.

The Avon Foundation's "Walk around the World for Breast Cancer" was held in several countries such as Guatemala, Germany, and United Arab Emirates. This walk seems to be less inundated with consumer products. However, the formula of corporate sponsorship used to fund the event is still in place. Logos of sponsors like Gatorade and New Balance are sprinkled throughout the walk itself (Avon Foundation 2008). The most common logo that is literally found on every banner, t-shirt, and balloon is Avon itself, which is of course a billion-dollar corporation that sells cosmetics to women in over one hundred countries.

For example, Avon's global efforts consist of organizing walks and fund-raisers in order to donate mammogram machines to countries all over the world and increase education about self-breast exam. According to the WHO, mammography is an extremely expensive test not available to women across the globe (WHO 2008). Yet the WHO specifically does not recommend focusing efforts on increasing the number of mammograms nor does it recommend self-screening. The WHO argues that encouraging women to get regular clinical screenings is far more effective. This tension represents a need for the organizations working on breast cancer at the global level to make an effort to coordinate better. The fact that Avon focuses on mammograms while the WHO focuses on clinical screenings indicates a need for a comprehensive and unified breast cancer activism. In addition, there are understandings of breast cancer that are being pushed aside by the discourses commonly used by the Komen and Avon foundations.

In the United States, cancer education and activism is a visual part of everyday life due to celebrities' speaking out, activist bracelets, books, and doctors' education. However, in other countries cancer is not something that is talked about publicly. Specifically, in China women do not speak of their breasts and therefore if they experience pain they are often extremely reluctant to discuss it even with their doctors. This habit of ignoring breast pain can lead to a fatal diagnosis of breast cancer. Even after diagnosis some Chinese women feel great shame and are reluctant to share their pain and news with family and others (Wong-Kim et al. 2005: 11). Also, some Chinese women often believe that breast cancer is payback from their ancestors or caused by their own immoral behavior, or accumulation of negative thoughts and feelings. (Wong-Kim et al. 2005: 9–10). Cultural beliefs about breast cancer are extremely important to know about, especially since China has one of the fastest growing breast cancer rates around the world (Avon Foundation 2008). Therefore for transnational feminist activism focused on breast cancer to be meaningful it must at least understand local cultural beliefs about the body and breast cancer. Metaphors used to understand the body and cancer can greatly vary across the globe. Therefore the danger is that as Avon and Komen foundations increase their efforts globally, metaphors, which are not universal, get exported as well. It is important that American metaphors for breast cancer are not pushed. It is equally as important not to substitute local cultural metaphors but rather challenge the way women with breast cancer are understood everywhere. Breast cancer is a leading cause of death for women around the world. It is important to participate in breast cancer activism in the hope that someday a cure will be found and in the meantime to help women deal with breast cancer. However, it is equally important to challenge mainstream modes of breast cancer activism and the narratives they advocate regarding women's bodies.

Notes

1. Notes for Dr. Susan Love's speech, NBCC Advocacy Training, Washington, DC, May 2011; in author's possession.

2. Anonymous, confidential phone interview by author, March 20, 2011; in author's possession.

3. Anonymous, confidential phone interview by author, December 17, 2010; in author's possession.

4. Anonymous, confidential interview by author, San Francisco, CA, February 8, 2011; in author's possession.

5. Anonymous, confidential phone interview by author, February 28, 2011; in author's possession.

6. Anonymous, confidential interview by author, San Francisco, MA, February 10, 2013; in author's possession.

7. Anonymous, confidential interview by author, Jamaica Plain, MA, November 5, 2010; in author's possession.

8. Anonymous, confidential interview by author, Boston, MA, November 17, 2010, in author's possession.

9. Anonymous, confidential interview by author, Boston, MA, November 17, 2010, in author's possession.

10. Anonymous, confidential interview by author, San Francisco, CA, February 11, 2011, in author's possession.

11. A qualitative approach also supports the use of emergent research design that enables the study to pursue research directions not anticipated prior to beginning the research (Creswell 2009: 135). In the early stages of this research, the pilot interviews were focused on individual preference for pink or green and factors that mobilize activists. It became clear that the research needed to be focused on organizations and their role in shaping pink or green advocacy. Therefore the interview questions were revised early on to focus on organizational attributes rather than individual motivations for activism. In other words, an emergent research design allowed me to pursue a research direction toward organizations that was not anticipated during the prospectus phase.

12. Anonymous, confidential interview by author, San Francisco, CA, February 10, 2011; in author's possession.

13. Anonymous, confidential interview by author, Boston, MA, March 11, 2011; in author's possession.

14. Anonymous and confidential interview by author, San Francisco, CA, February 11, 2011, in author's possession.

15. Anonymous, confidential interview by author, San Francisco, CA, February 8, 2011; in author's possession.

Appendix A: Acronyms

ACS	American Cancer Society
BCA	Breast Cancer Action
BCC	Breast Cancer Connections
BCF	Breast Cancer Fund
BRCA1/BRCA2	Breast Cancer Gene Mutation
CDC	Centers for Disease Control and Prevention
DOD	Department of Defense
DPH	Department of Public Health
EPA	Environmental Protection Agency
EWG	Environmental Working Group
FDA	Food and Drug Administration
MBCC	Massachusetts Breast Cancer Coalition
NABCO	National Alliance of Breast Cancer Organizations
NBCAM	National Breast Cancer Awareness Month
NBCC	National Breast Cancer Coalition
NCI	National Cancer Institute
NIH	National Institutes of Health
NSF	National Science Foundation
Project LEAD	Leadership, Education, and Advocacy Development
TSCA	Toxic Substances Control Act
WFA	Women's Field Army
YSC	Young Survival Coalition

Appendix B: Time Line

1882   Halsted develops radical mastectomy

1913   American Society for the Control of Cancer is founded

1936   Society for the Control of Cancer forms Women's Field Army

1955   Avon Foundation founded

1962   Rachel Carson publishes *Silent Spring*

1970   U.S. Environmental Protection Agency established

1973   *Our Bodies Our Selves* published by the Boston Women's Health Collective

1974   Betty Ford publicly reveals her breast cancer diagnosis

1975   Rose Kushner establishes Breast Cancer Advisory Center

1976   Toxic Substances Control Act (TSCA)

1978   Love Canal of Niagara Falls, New York, evacuated after protests of high cancer rates and birth defects due to toxic chemicals buried under homes and schools

1978   Y-ME founded

1978   Susan Sontag publishes *Illness as Metaphor*

1980   Audre Lorde publishes *The Cancer Journals*

1982   Warren County, North Carolina, protests hazardous waste landfill and PCBs polluting drinking water

1982   Rose Kushner publishes *What Every Woman Should Know about Breast Cancer to Save Her Life*

1982   Nancy Brinker founds Susan G. Komen for the Cure

1984   DES linked to breast cancer

1985   National Breast Cancer Awareness Month (NBCAM) established by ACS

1986   NABCO founded

1987   ACT UP founded

1989   Montini and Ruzek publish "Overturning Orthodoxy: The Emergence of Breast Cancer Treatment Policy"

1990   Breast Cancer Action forms and publicly criticizes ACS for focus on cure and treatment only

1990   Breast and Cervical Cancer Mortality Prevention Act

1990   The Mautner Project founded

1990   Komen Foundation hands out pink visors at Race for the Cure

1991   Komen hands out pink ribbons at NYC race

1991   Bush administration forms President's Commission on Breast Cancer

1991   National Breast Cancer Coalition forms and its Massachusetts Chapter

1992   Precautionary Principle defined in the Rio Declaration on Environment and Development

1992   Breast Cancer Help, Inc. founded

1992   Breast Cancer Fund founded

1992   Pink ribbon becomes official symbol for NBCAM

1993   Department of Defense Peer-Reviewed Breast Cancer Research Program

1993   Long Island Breast Cancer Study

1993   Avon holds "Crusade for the Cure"

1993   Matuschka is on the cover of *New York Times Magazine* with mastectomy scar

1993	President Clinton creates National Mammography Day in October
1993	Breast Cancer Research Foundation founded
1993	BRCA1 gene identified
1994	Toxic Links Coalition founded
1994	Silent Spring Institute founded
1995	Marin Breast Cancer Watch founded
1995	BRCA2 gene identified
1996	Roberta Altman publishes *Waking Up Fighting Back*
1997	Balanced Budget Act expands Medicare mammography coverage
1997	Stamp Out Breast Cancer Act
1997	Steingraber publishes *Living Downstream*
1998	Avon holds 3-day walk for breast cancer, which is criticized by BCA
1998	BCA places ad in *New York Times* "Who's Really Cleaning Up?"
1998	Young Survival Coalition founded
1999	NOW asks for more funding for research into the causes of breast cancer
1999	Ellen Leopold publishes *A Darker Ribbon*
2000	Laura Potts publishes *Ideologies of Breast Cancer*
2000	BCA launches "Think Twice before You Walk Campaign"
2000	Kasper and Ferguson publish *A Society Shapes an Epidemic*
2001	Casamayou publishes *Politics of Breast Cancer*
2001	Barbara Ehrenreich publishes "Welcome to Cancer Land"
2001	BCA launches "Think before You Pink Campaign"
2004	NABCO disbands
2004	Samantha King publishes *Pink Ribbons, Inc.*
2005	Marin Breast Cancer Watch becomes Zero Breast Cancer
2007	Komen and Silent Spring Institute publish *Environmental Factors in Breast Cancer*

2007   Komen Foundation changes its name to Susan G. Komen for the Cure

2008   Klawiter publishes *The Biopolitics of Breast Cancer*

2008   President's Cancer Panel investigates environmental cancer risk

2008   Komen supports the Breast Cancer and Environmental Research Act

2009   Ley publishes *From Pink to Green*

2010   Komen invests in the Institute of Medicine to review scientific evidence on environment and cancer

2010   NBCC launches Breast Cancer Deadline 2020

2011   Komen announces BPA statement

2011   Komen asks Institute of Medicine to review scientific evidence on breast cancer and environment

2012   Komen defunds Planned Parenthood and then reinstates funding

Appendix C: Organizations

Breast Cancer Action
657 Mission Street, Suite 302
San Francisco, California 94105
(P) 415-243-9301

Breast Cancer Fund
388 Sutter Street, Suite 400
San Francisco, California 94109-5400
(P) 415-346-8223

National Breast Cancer Coalition
1010 Vermont Avenue, NW, Suite 900
Washington, DC 2005
    Massachusetts Breast Cancer Coalition
    Post Office Box 222
    Rockland, Massachusetts 02370
    (P) 617-376-6222

Susan G. Komen 5005 LBJ Freeway Suite 250
    Dallas, Texas
    (P) 1-877-GO KOMEN
    Susan G. Komen Massachusetts
    200 Brickstone Square, Suite 407
    Andover, Massachusetts 01810
    (P) 978-409-1859

Avon Foundation Breast Cancer Crusade
777 Third Avenue
New York, New York 10017
    (P) 866-505-AVON

Zero Breast Cancer
4340 Redwood Hwy
Suite C400
San Rafael, California 94903
(P) 415-507-1645

References

Chapter 1

Altman, R. (1996). *Waking up: Fighting back*. Boston, MA: Little Brown & Co.

American Cancer Society. (2014). *Cancer facts and figures 2012*. Retrieved March 2, 2015, from http://www.cancer.org/research/cancerfacts statistics/cancerfactsfigures2012/.

Andrews, K., & Edwards, B. (2004). Advocacy organizations in the U.S. political process. *Annual Review of Sociology, 30*, 479–506.

Avon Foundation. (2013). *Avon Foundation for Women 2013 audited results—Topline financial summary*. http://www.avonfoundation. org/assets/2014/2013-avon-foundation-topline-financial-summary. pdf (Accessed on March 11, 2015).

Blee, K., & Taylor, V. (2002). Semi-structured interviewing in social movement research. In B. Klandermas & S. Staggenborg (Eds.), *Methods of social movement research*. Minneapolis: University of Minnesota Press, 92–117.

Boehmer, U. (2000). *The personal and political*. Albany: State University of New York Press.

Braun, L. (2003). Engaging the experts: Popular science education and breast cancer activism. *Critical Public Health, 13*(3), 191–195.

Breast Cancer Fund. (2015). Retrieved July 20, 2015, from www.breast cancerfund.org

Brenner, B. (2012). Interview by Zaylia A. Pluss in San Francisco, CA. Accessed through Sophia Smith Collection, Smith College 2012.

Brown, P. (2007). *Toxic exposures*. New York: Columbia University Press.

Brown, P., Zavestoski, S., McCormick, S., Mayer, B., Morello-Frosch, R., & Altman, R. G. (2004). Embodied health movements: New approaches to social movements in health. *Sociology of Health & Illness, 26*(1), 50–80.

Bullard, R. (1990). *Dumping in Dixie: Race, class, and environmental quality.* Boulder, CO: Westview.

California Breast Cancer Research Program (CBCRP). (2007). *Identifying gaps in breast cancer research.* Retrieved from http:www.cbcrp.org

Carson, R. (1994). *Silent spring: With an introduction by Al Gore.* Boston, MA: Houghton.

Creswell, J. (2009). *Research design: Qualitative, quantitative and mixed methods.* Thousand Oaks, CA: Sage.

Ehrenreich, B. (2001). Welcome to cancerland: A mammogram leads to a cult of pink kitsch. *Harper's Magazine,* 47.

Kedrowski, K., & Sarow, M. S. (2007). *Cancer activism.* Chicago: University of Illinois Press.

King, S. (2004). Pink Ribbons, Inc.: Breast cancer activism and the politics of philanthropy. *International Journal of Qualitative Studies in Education (QSE),* 17, 473–492.

King, S. (2008). *Pink Ribbons, Inc.: Breast cancer and the politics of philanthropy.* Minneapolis: University of Minnesota Press.

Klawiter, M. (2008). *The biopolitics of breast cancer.* Minneapolis: University of Minnesota Press.

Leopold, E. (1999). *A darker ribbon: Breast cancer, women, and their doctors in the twentieth century.* Boston, MA: Beacon Press.

Ley, B. L. (2009). *From pink to green.* New Brunswick, NJ: Rutgers University Press.

Massachusetts Breast Cancer Coalition. (2015). www.mbcc.org

McCormick, S. (2009). *Mobilizing science.* Philadelphia, PA: Temple University Press.

McCormick, S. (2010). *No family history.* Lanham, MD: Rowman and Littlefield.

Miles, M., & Huberman, M. (Eds.). (1994). *Qualitative data analysis.* Thousand Oaks, CA: Sage.

Montini, T., & Ruzek, S. (1989). Overturning orthodoxy: The emergence of breast cancer treatment policy. *Research in Sociology of Health Care,* 8, 3–32.

National Breast Cancer Coalition. (2011–2012). Organizational materials provided prior to and during Advocacy Training Conference in May in Washington, DC.

National Cancer Institute. (2008–2009). *Environmental factors in cancer.* Washington, DC: President's Cancer Panel, National Cancer Institute [Online]. http://deainfo.nci.nih.gov/advisory/pcp/annualReports/index.htm (Accessed on January 6, 2013).

Neuman, W. L. (2006). *Social research methods* (6th ed.). Boston, MA: University of Wisconsin at Whitewater.

Potts, L. K. (2000). *Ideologies of breast cancer: Feminist perspectives.* London: Palgrave Macmillan.

Silent Spring Institute. (2015). *Body burden.* www.http://www.silentspring .org/body-burden (Accessed February 28, 2015).

Silent Spring Institute. (2007). *Environmental Factors in Breast Cancer* from www.silentspring.org.

Sulik, G. (2012). *Pink ribbon blues: How breast cancer culture undermines women's health.* Oxford: Oxford University Press.

Chapter 2

Anderson, W. (2004). We can do it: A study of the Women's Field Army public relations efforts. *Public Relations Review, 30*(2), 187–196.

Avon Foundation. (2011a). *Early detection saves lives: Breast Health Resource Guide.* http://www.avonfoundation.org/assets/bccguide.pdf

Avon Foundation. (2011b). Where the money goes. Promotional handout given at 2008 walk.

Avon Foundation. (2008–2011). The Avon Breast Cancer Crusade. Promotional handout given at meetings in Boston and San Francisco.

Barakso, M. (2010). Brand identity and the tactical repertoires of advocacy organizations. In A. Prakash & M. K. Gugerty (Eds.), *Advocacy organizations and collective action* (pp. 155–176). Cambridge: Cambridge University Press.

Benford, R., & Snow, D. (2000). Framing processes and social movements: An overview and assessment. *Annual Review of Sociology, 26,* 611–639.

Bloodgood, E. (2010). Institutional environment and the organization of advocacy NGOs in the OECD. In A. Prakash & M. K. Gugerty (Eds.), *Advocacy organizations and collective action* (pp. 91–130). Cambridge: Cambridge University Press.

Bosso, C. (2003). Rethinking the Concept of Membership in Nature Advocacy Organizations. *Policy Studies Journal, 31*(3), 397–411.

Boston Women's Health Book, & J. Norsigian Collective. (2011). *Our bodies ourselves* (40 Anv. ed.). Touchstone.

Breast Cancer Fund. (2011, February). Breast Cancer Fund's Event. Speech by Jeanne Rizzo. San Francisco, CA.

Breast Cancer Fund and the Collaborative on Health and the Environment. (2010). Highlights from the President's Cancer Panel *Reducing Environmental Cancer Risk* Report. http://www.breastcancerfund .org/assets/pdfs/tips-fact-sheets/presidents-cancer-panel-fact.pdf

Brenner, B. (2012). Interview by Zaylia A. Pluss in San Francisco, CA. Accessed through Sophia Smith Collection, Smith College 2012.

Brenner, B. (2002). *Exercise your mind,* Breast Cancer Action, Newsletter 58, March/April, 2000, http://www.bcaction.org/Pages/Searchable Pages/2000Newsletters/Newsletter058B.html

Brown, P. (2007). *Toxic exposures.* New York: Columbia University Press.

Bullard, R. (1990). *Dumping in Dixie: Race, class, and environmental quality.* Boulder, CO: Westview.

Carson, R. (1994). *Silent spring: With an introduction by Al Gore.* Boston, MA: Houghton.

Conrad, P., & Leiter, V. (2003). *Health and health care as social problems.* Boston, MA: Rowman and Littlefield.

Feinstein, D. (2015). *Feinstein, Enzi introduce bill to reauthorize breast cancer research stamp.* http://www.feinstein.senate.gov/public/index. cfm/press-releases?ID=9235c3db-9bd9-4456-8583-a1ca4e3192a0

Gerber, E. (1999). *The populist paradox: Interest group influence and the promise of direct legislation.* Princeton, NJ: Princeton University Press.

Goffman, E. (1974). *Frame analysis: An essay on the organization of experience.* New York: Harper & Row.

Institute of Medicine. (2011). *Breast cancer and the environment: A life course approach* [Online]. http://www.iom.edu/Reports/2011/Breast -Cancer-and-the-Environment-A-Life-Course-Approach.aspx (Accessed June 2011).

Kasper, A. S., & Ferguson, S. (2000). *Breast cancer.* New York: Palgrave Macmillan.

Kedrowski, K., & Sarow, M. S. (2007). *Cancer activism.* Chicago: University of Illinois Press.

King, S. (2004). Pink ribbons Inc.: Breast cancer activism and the politics of philanthropy. *International Journal of Qualitative Studies in Education (QSE), 17,* 473–492.

King, S. (2008). *Pink Ribbons, Inc.: Breast cancer and the politics of philanthropy.* Minneapolis: University of Minnesota Press.

Klawiter, M. (2008). *The biopolitics of breast cancer.* Minneapolis: University of Minnesota Press.

Kolker, E. S. (2004). Framing as a cultural resource in health social movements: Funding activism and the breast cancer movement in the US 1990–1993. *Sociology of Health & Illness, 26,* 820–844.

Komen Foundation. (2009). Advocacy Alliance. http://ww5.komen.org/ GetInvolved/kaa.html

Komen Foundation. (2011). *You Can Do This.* Promotional materials sent in the mail.

Komen Foundation. (2012). Massachusetts. About Us. http://www.komen mass.org/site/c.6oIEJTPxGcISF/b.8708397/k.C987/About_Us.htm

Kushner, R. (1982). *Why me? What every woman should know about breast cancer.* New York: Henry Holt & Co.

Ley, B. L. (2009). *From pink to green.* New Brunswick, NJ: Rutgers University Press.

Lorde, A. (2006). *The cancer journals.* Special edition. San Francisco, CA: Aunt Lute Books.

Massachusetts Breast Cancer Coalition. (2015). www.mbcc.org.

McAdam, D., & Snow, D. (Eds.). (2010). *Readings on social movements.* Oxford, UK: Oxford University Press.

McCormick, S. (2009). *Mobilizing science.* Philadelphia, PA: Temple University Press.

National Breast Cancer Coalition. (2011–2012). Introductory Letter and Organizational materials collected at the NBCC Annual Advocacy Training Conference held May 2011 in Washington, DC.

National Breast Cancer Coalition. (2011). Guide to the 112th Congress National Breast Cancer Coalition. Distributed at the NBCC Annual Advocacy Training Conference held May 2011 in Washington, DC.

National Cancer Institute. (2008–2009). *Environmental factors in cancer.* Washington, DC: President's Cancer Panel, National Cancer Institute [Online]. http://deainfo.nci.nih.gov/advisory/pcp/annualReports/index.htm (Accessed January 6, 2013).

Parthasarathy, S. (2010). Breaking the expertise barrier: Understanding activist strategies in science and technology policy domains. *Science and Public Policy, 37,* 355–367.

Patel, K., & Rushefsky, M. (2005). *The politics of public health in the United States.* Armank, NY: M.E. Sharpe.

Prakash, A., & Gugerty, M. K. (Eds.). (2010). *Advocacy organizations and collective action.* New York: Cambridge University Press.

Silent Spring Institute. (2010, February 1). *Cape Cod breast cancer and environment study.* Retrieved from www.silentspring.org.

Snow, D., & Benford, R. (1988). Ideology, frame resonance, and participant mobilization. *International Social Movement Research, 1,* 197–217.

Snow, D., Rochford, E. B., Worden, S. K., & Benford, R. D. (1986). Frame alignment processes, micromobilization, and movement participation. *American Sociological Review, 51,* 464–481.

Steingraber, S. (1997a). Mechanisms, proof, and unmet needs: The perspective of a cancer activist. *Environmental Health Perspectives, 105,* 685–687.

Steingraber, S. (1997b). *Living down stream.* Reading, MA: Wesley.

Sulik, G. (2012). *Pink ribbon blues: How breast cancer culture undermines women's health.* Oxford: Oxford University Press.

Swissler, M. (2003). Compromised? The Susan G. Komen Foundation is tied up in private interests that run counter to its mission. *Creative Loafing, 17,* 30–39.

Turshen, M. (2007). *Women's health movements: A global force for change.* New York: Palgrave Macmillan.

Wailoo, K. (2011). *How cancer crossed the color line.* Oxford: Oxford University Press.

Weisman, C. S. (2000). Breast cancer policymaking. In A. S. Kasper & J. S. Ferguson (Eds.), *Breast cancer: Society shapes an epidemic* (pp. 213–244). New York: St. Martin's Press.

Young, M. (2010). In A. Prakash & M. K. Gugerty (Eds.), *Advocacy organizations and collective action*. New York: Cambridge University Press.

Chapter 3

Anglin, M. K. (1997). Working from the inside out: Implications of breast cancer activism for biomedical policies and practices. *Social Science & Medicine, 44*, 1403–1415.

Braun, L. (2003). Engaging the experts: Popular science education and breast cancer activism. *Critical Public Health, 13*(3), 191–195.

Breast Cancer Action. (2014a). *Don't frack with our health*. http://www.bcaction.org/take-action/stop-fracking/

Breast Cancer Action. (2014b). *Why fracking must be banned by Sandra Steingraber*. http://bcaction.org/2012/11/01/why-fracking-must-be-banned/

Breast Cancer Action. (2014c). *What the frack? Drill rig goes pink(washing) for breast cancer by Annie Sartor*. http://bcaction.org/2012/11/15/what-the-frack-drill-rig-goes-pinkwashing-for-breast-cancer/

Breast Cancer Fund. (2010). *State of the evidence: The connection between breast cancer and the environment by Janet Gray, Ph.D.* Retrieved March 2, 2015, from http://www.breastcancerfund.org/assets/pdfs/publications/state-of-the-evidence-2010.pdf

Breast Cancer Fund. (2015). *About the Breast Cancer Fund*. http://www.breastcancerfund.org/about/

Breast Cancer Fund. (2014). *Support full disclosure of fracking chemicals*. https://secure3.convio.net/bcf/site/Advocacy?cmd=display&page=UserAction&id=241

Breast Cancer Fund. (2010). *State of the Evidence*. http://www.breastcancerfund.org/media/publications/state-of-the-evidence/

Brody, J. G., Tickner, J., & Rudel, R. A. (2005). Community initiated breast cancer and environment studies and the precautionary principle. *Environmental Health Perspectives, 113*, 920–925.

Brown, P. (2007). *Toxic exposures*. New York: Columbia University Press.

Cassamayou, M. (2001). *The politics of breast cancer*. Washington, DC: Georgetown University Press.

Committee on Energy & Commerce, Democrats. (2011). *Committee democrats release new report detailing hydraulic fracturing products*. http://democrats.energycommerce.house.gov/index.php?q=news/committee-democrats-release-new-report-detailing-hydraulic-fracturing-products

Conrad, P., & Leiter, V. (2003). *Health and health care as social problems*. Boston, MA: Rowman and Littlefield.

Environmental Protection Agency. (2014a). *Natural gas extraction-hydraulic fracturing*. http://www2.epa.gov/hydraulicfracturing

Environmental Protection Agency. (2014b). *Endocrine disruptor research initiative, fact sheet.* http://www.epa.gov/edrlupvx/edrifact.html

Environmental Protection Agency. (2012a). *Benzene.* http://www.epa.gov/ttn/atw/hlthef/benzene.html

Environmental Protection Agency. (2012b). *Toluene.* http://www.epa.gov/ttn/atw/hlthef/toluene.html

Environmental Working Group. (2009). *Pollution in minority newborns: BPA and other cord blood pollutants.* Retrieved from www.ewg.org

Food and Water Watch. (2013). *The social costs of fracking.* http://documents.foodandwaterwatch.org/doc/Social_Costs_of_Fracking.pdf

Institute of Medicine. (2011). *Breast cancer and the environment: A life course approach* [Online]. http://www.iom.edu/Reports/2011/Breast-Cancer-and-the-Environment-A-Life-Course-Approach.aspx (Accessed June 2011).

Institute of Medicine. (2011). *IOM report identifies steps that may reduce women's risk for breast cancer associated with environmental factors.* http://www.iom.edu/Reports/2011/Breast-Cancer-and-the-Environment-A-Life-Course-Approach/Press-Release.aspx

Komen Foundation. (2010, October 22). *Susan G. Komen for the Cure BPA Statement.* https://ww5.komen.org/uploadedFiles/Content_Binaries/BPAStatementOctober2011.pdf

Komen Foundation. (2010). Circle of promise campaign. Retrieved from http://www.komen.org

Komen Foundation. (2011, October 22). *Susan G. Komen for the Cure BPA Statement.* https://ww5.komen.org/uploadedFiles/Content_Binaries/BPAStatementOctober2011.pdf

Lerner, B. (2001). *Breast cancer wars.* London, UK: Oxford University Press.

Ley, B. L. (2009). *From pink to green.* New Brunswick, NJ: Rutgers University Press.

McCormick, S. (2009). *Mobilizing science.* Philadelphia, PA: Temple University Press.

McDermott-Levy, R., Kaktins, N., & Sattler, B. (2013). Fracking, the environment, and health: New energy practices may threaten public health. *American Journal of Nursing, 113*(6), 45–51.

National Breast Cancer Coalition. (2011–2012). Introductory Letter and Organizational materials collected at the NBCC Annual Advocacy Training Conference held May 2011 in Washington, DC.

National Breast Cancer Coalition. (2015). *About NBCC.* http://www.breastcancerdeadline2020.org/about-nbcc/

National Cancer Institute. (2008–2009). *Environmental factors in cancer.* Washington, DC: President's Cancer Panel, National Cancer Institute [Online]. http://deainfo.nci.nih.gov/advisory/pcp/annualReports/index.htm (Accessed January 6, 2013).

National Cancer Institute. (2008). *Questions and answers about the breast cancer and the environment on long island study.* Retrieved March 2, 2015, from http://www.cancer.gov/newscenter/qa/2002/long-island -environmentqa

Schonfelder, G., Wittoht, W., Hopp, H., Talsness, C. E., Paul, M., & Chahoud, I. (2002). Parent bisphenol A accumulation in the human maternal-fetal-placental unit. *Environmental Health Perspective, 110*(11), A703–A707.

Steingraber, S. (1997a). Mechanisms, proof, and unmet needs: The perspective of a cancer activist. *Environmental Health Perspectives, 105,* 685–687.

Steingraber, S. (1997b). *Living down stream.* Reading, MA: Wesley.

Chapter 4

American Cancer Society. (2015). *Cancer facts and figures 2015.* Retrieved March 2, 2015, from http://www.cancer.org/research/cancerfacts statistics/cancerfactsfigures2015/index

Atlantic.com. (2012). *Top official at Susan G. Komen resigned over planned parenthood cave in.* Retrieved from http://www.theatlantic.com/ health/archive/2012/02/top-susan-g-komen-official-resigned-over -planned-parenthood-cave-in/252405/

Avon Foundation. *Avon walk videos.* May 16, 2007, from http://walk .avonfoundation.org

Avon Foundation. *Why walk.* May 16, 2007, from http://walk.avon foundation.org

Barakso, M. (2010). Brand identity and the tactical repertoires of advocacy organizations. In A. Prakash & M. K. Gugerty (Eds.), *Advocacy organizations and collective action* (pp. 155–176). Cambridge: Cambridge University Press.

Birke, L. (1998). "Bodies and Biology." From "Biological Sciences." In A. Jagger & I. Young (Eds.), *Companion to feminist philosophy.* Oxford: Blackwell, 42–49.

Breast Cancer Action. (2012a). *Turning knowledge into action.* Webinar presented by Sahru Keiser, MPH.

Breast Cancer Action. (2010b). Retrieved from www.bca.org

Breast Cancer Action. (2014c). *What the frack? Drill rig goes pinkwashing for breast cancer by Annie Sartor.* http://bcaction.org/2012/11/15/ what-the-frack-drill-rig-goes-pinkwashing-for-breast-cancer/

Breast Cancer Action. (2015d). *Annual Summary 2010–2011.* http://www .bcaction.org/about/annual-summary/

Breast Cancer Fund. (2015). *Pink Ribbons, Fracking Drill Bits and Football.* http://www.breastcancerfund.org/media/press-releases/fracking.html

Brenner, B. (2012). Interview by Zaylia A. Pluss in San Francisco, CA. Accessed through Sophia Smith Collection, Smith College 2012.

Eisenstein, Z. (2001). *Manmade breast cancer*. Ithaca, NY: Cornell University Press.

Elliott, C. (2007). Pink!: Community, contestation, and the color of breast cancer. *Canadian Journal of Communication, 32*, 521–536.

Ford. *Calling all warriors*. May 17, 2007, from http://www.fordvehicles .com/warriorsinpink/wip/

Hughes, B. (2015). *Baker Hughes Supports Susan G. Komen's mission to end breast cancer forever*. http://public.bakerhughes.com/pink/ (Accessed March 30, 2015).

Kasper, A. S., & Ferguson, S. (2000). *Breast cancer*. New York: Palgrave Macmillan.

King, S. (2008). *Pink Ribbons, Inc.: Breast cancer and the politics of philanthropy*. Minneapolis: University of Minnesota Press.

Klawiter, M. (2008). *The biopolitics of breast cancer*. Minneapolis: University of Minnesota Press.

Komen Foundation. *How funds are used*. November 30, 2006, from http:// www.komen.org/intradoc-cgi/idc_cgi_isapi.dll?IdcService=SS_GET _PAGE&nodeId=525

Leopold, E. (1999). *A darker ribbon: Breast cancer, women, and their doctors in the twentieth century*. Boston, MA: Beacon Press.

Lerner, B. (2001). *Breast cancer wars*. London, UK: Oxford University Press.

Ley, B. L. (2009). *From pink to green*. New Brunswick, NJ: Rutgers University Press.

Lupton, D. (1994). The body in medicine. In *Medicine as culture. Illness disease and the body in western society*. London: Sage Publications.

Martin, E. (1999). The egg and the sperm: How science has constructed a romance based on stereotypical male-female roles. In J. Price & M. Shildrick (Eds.), *Feminist theory and the body: A reader* (pp. 179–189). New York: Routledge.

Martin, E. (1998). The fetus as intruder. In R. Davis-Floyd & J. Dumit (Eds.), *Cyborg babies*. New York: Routledge.

Mayer, M. (1998). *Advanced breast cancer: A guide to living with metastatic disease*. Beijing: O'Reilly Media Inc.

McClintock, A. (1996). No longer in a future heaven: Nationalism, gender, and race. In G. Eley & R. G. Suny (Eds.), *Becoming national: A reader* (pp. 260–284). New York: Oxford University Press.

McCormick, S. (2009). *Mobilizing science*. Philadelphia, PA: Temple University Press.

National Breast Cancer Awareness Month. November 30, 2006, from http:// www.whitehouse.gov/news/releases/2005/09/20050930-10.html

Prakash, A., & Gugerty, M. K. (Eds.). (2010). *Advocacy organizations and collective action*. New York: Cambridge University Press.

Sedgwick, E. K. (1999). Breast cancer: An adventure in applied deconstruction. In J. Price & M. Schildrick (Eds.), *Feminist theory and the body: A reader*. New York: Routledge, 153–156.

Sontag, S. (2001). *Illness as metaphor*. New York: Picador.

Stacey, J. (1997). *Teratologies: A cultural study of cancer*. London: Routledge.

Sulik, G. (2012). *Pink Ribbon Blues: How breast cancer culture undermines women's health*. Oxford: Oxford University Press.

Visco, Fran. (2012). "Breast Cancer Deadline 2020." National Breast Cancer Coalition.

Warrior Women. Retrieved May 16, 2007, from http://www.ibcpatients.org/.

Young, I. (2005). Breasted Experience. In *On Female Body Experience: 'Throwing like a girl and other essays'*. Oxford University Press.

Chapter 5

Andrews, K., & Edwards, B. (2004). Advocacy organizations in the U.S. political process. *Annual Review of Sociology, 30*, 479–506.

Avon Foundation. *Avon walk videos*. May 16, 2007, from http://walk.avonfoundation.org

Avon Foundation. June 29, 2008, from http://info.avonfoundation.org/site/PageServer?pagename=waw_video

Army of Women (2011, March). *In Honor of Women's History Month*. Email sent to members.

Barakso, M. (2010). Brand identity and the tactical repertoires of advocacy organizations. In A. Prakash & M. K. Gugerty (Eds.), *Advocacy organizations and collective action* (pp. 155–176). Cambridge: Cambridge University Press.

Boehmer, U. (2000). *The personal and political*. Albany: State University of New York Press.

Braun, L. (2003). Engaging the experts: Popular science education and breast cancer activism. *Critical Public Health, 13*(3), 191–195.

Brendtro, M. J. (1998). Breast cancer: Agenda setting through activism. *Advanced Practice Nursing Quarterly, 4*(1), 54–63.

Brown, P. (2007). *Toxic exposures*. New York: Columbia University Press.

Brown, P., & Zayetoski, S. (2005). *Social movements in health*. Malden, MA: Blackwell.

Brown, P., Zavestoski, S., McCormick, S., Mayer, B., Morello-Frosch, R., & Altman, R. G. (2004). Embodied health movements: New approaches to social movements in health. *Sociology of Health & Illness, 26*(1), 50–80.

Creswell, J. (2009). *Research design: Qualitative, quantitative and mixed methods*. Thousand Oaks, CA: Sage.

Earp, J., French, E., & Gilkey, M. (2008). *Patient advocacy for health care quality*. Sudbury, MA: Jones and Bartlett Publishers.

Heaney, M., & McClurg, S. (2009). Social networks and American politics: Introduction to the special issue. *American Politics Research, 37*, 727.

Ireland, P. (1999). Make Breast Cancer Prevention a Priority Issue in 2000. National Organization for Women. http://www.now.org/cgi-bin/search .cgi?fmt=long&form=extended&m=all&np=18&ps=10&q=breast &s=RPD&sp=1&ul=&wm=end

Jenkins, J. C. (1987). Nonprofit organizations and political advocacy. In W. Powell (Ed.), *The nonprofit sector: A research handbook* (pp. 296–320). New Haven, CT: Yale University Press.

Karbon, R. (2010). Does Sharing your Bra Color Equal Breast Cancer Awareness? National Organization for Women, Blog for Equality. http://now.org/blog/does-sharing-your-bra-color-equal-breast-cancer -awareness/

King, S. (2008). *Pink Ribbons, Inc.: Breast cancer and the politics of philanthropy*. Minneapolis: University of Minnesota Press.

Klawiter, M. (2008). *The biopolitics of breast cancer*. Minneapolis: University of Minnesota Press.

Knoke, D., & Yang, S. (2008). *Social network analysis*. Thousand Oaks, CA: Sage.

Komen Foundation. (2012). *Advocacy Alliance*. http://ww5.komen.org/ GetInvolved/kaa.html

Komen Foundation. (2010). *Circle of promise campaign*. Retrieved from http://www.komen.org

Komen Foundation. (2007). We're looking for some women to work around the house. *Organizational material*.

McCormick, S. (2009). *Mobilizing science*. Philadelphia, PA: Temple University Press.

Meyer, D. S., & Whittier, N. (1994). Social movement spillover. *Social Problems, 41*, 277–298.

Mitchell, J. C. (1969). The concept and use of social networks. In J. C. Mitchell (Ed.), *Social networks in urban situations* (pp. 1–50). Manchester: Manchester University Press.

National Cancer Institute. (2010). Retrieved from www.nci.org

National Organization for Women. (2000). *NOW Unites with Breast Cancer Groups for Research on Causes and Prevention*. http://www .now.org/cgi-bin/search.cgi?fmt=long&form=extended&m=all&np=13 &ps=20&q=breast&s=RPD&sp=1&su=title&ul=&wm=wrd

Prakash, A., & Gugerty, M. K. (Eds.). (2010). *Advocacy organizations and collective action*. New York: Cambridge University Press.

Stein, R. (2004). *New perspectives on environmental justice*. New Brunswick, NJ: Rutgers University Press.

Strolovich, D. Z. (2007). *Affirmative advocacy: Race, class, and gender in interest group politics*. Chicago, IL: University of Chicago Press.

Turshen, M. (2007). *Women's health movements: A global force for change.* New York: Palgrave Macmillan.

Wong-Kim, E., Sun, A., & DeMattos, M. (2003). Assessing cancer beliefs in a Chinese immigrant community. *Cancer Control, 10,* 22–28.

World Health Organization. (2008a). *Cancer.* http://www.who.int/mediacentre/factsheets/fs297/en/index.html

World Health Organization. (2008b). *Screening for breast cancer.* http://www.who.int/cancer/detection/breastcancer/en/

COMPLETE LIST OF REFERENCES

Altman, R. (1996). *Waking up: Fighting back.* Boston, MA: Little Brown & Co.

American Cancer Society. (2015). *Cancer facts and figures 2015.* Retrieved March 2, 2015, from http://www.cancer.org/research/cancerfacts statistics/cancerfactsfigures2015/index

American Cancer Society. (2012). Cancer facts and figures 2012. Retrieved March 2, 2015, from http://www.cancer.org/research/cancerfacts statistics/cancerfactsfigures2012/

Anderson, W. (2004). We can do it: A study of the Women's Field Army public relations efforts. *Public Relations Review, 30*(2), 187–196.

Andrews, K., & Edwards, B. (2004). Advocacy organizations in the U.S. political process. *Annual Review of Sociology, 30,* 479–506.

Anglin, M. K. (1997). Working from the inside out: Implications of breast cancer activism for biomedical policies and practices. *Social Science & Medicine, 44,* 1403–1415.

Atlantic.com. (2012). *Top official at Susan G. Komen resigned over planned parenthood cave in.* Retrieved from http://www.theatlantic.com/health/archive/2012/02/top-susan-g-komen-official-resigned-over-planned-parenthood-cave-in/252405/

Avon. (2013). *Avon Foundation for Women 2013 audited results – Topline financial summary.* http://www.avonfoundation.org/assets/2014/2013-avon-foundation-topline-financial-summary.pdf (Accessed March 11, 2015).

Avon Foundation. *Avon walk videos.* May 16, 2007, from http://walk.avonfoundation.org

Avon Foundation. *Why walk.* May 16, 2007, from http://walk.avonfoundation.org

Avon Foundation. June 29, 2008, from http://info.avonfoundation.org/site/PageServer?pagename=waw_video

Avon Walk for Breast Cancer. Washington, DC. November 30, 2006, from http://walk.avonfoundation.org/site/DocServer/4.30.06_DC_CLOSING_FINAL.pdf?docID=4462

Barakso, M. (2010). Brand identity and the tactical repertoires of advocacy organizations. In A. Prakash & M. K. Gugerty (Eds.), *Advocacy organizations and collective action* (pp. 155–176). Cambridge: Cambridge University Press.

Benford, R., & Snow, D. (2000). Framing processes and social movements: An overview and assessment. *Annual Review of Sociology, 26,* 611–639.

Birke, L. (1998). "Bodies and Biology." From "Biological Sciences." In A. Jagger & I. Young (Eds.), *Companion to feminist philosophy.* Oxford: Blackwell, 42–49.

Bloodgood, E. (2010). Institutional environment and the organization of advocacy NGOs in the OECD. In A. Prakash & M. K. Gugerty (Eds.), *Advocacy organizations and collective action* (pp. 91–130). Cambridge: Cambridge University Press.

Boehmer, U. (2000). *The personal and political.* Albany: State University of New York Press.

Bosso, C. J. (1988). *Pesticides and politics: The life cycle of public issue.* Pittsburgh, PA: University of Pittsburgh Press.

Boston Women's Health Book, & J. Norsigian Collective. (2011). *Our bodies ourselves* (40 Anv. ed.). Touchstone.

Braun, L. (2003). Engaging the experts: Popular science education and breast cancer activism. *Critical Public Health, 13*(3), 191–195.

Breast Cancer Action. (2012). *Turning knowledge into action.* Webinar presented by Sahru Keiser, MPH.

Breast Cancer Action. (2010). Retrieved from www.bca.org

Breast Cancer Action. *Where does the pink ribbon come from?* December 17, 2006, from www.bcaction.org

Breast Cancer Action. (2014a). *Don't frack with our health.* http://www.bcaction.org/take-action/stop-fracking/

Breast Cancer Action. (2014b). *Why fracking must be banned by Sandra Steingraber.* http://bcaction.org/2012/11/01/why-fracking-must-be-banned/

Breast Cancer Action. (2014c). *What the frack? Drill rig goes pinkwashing for breast cancer by Annie Sartor.* http://bcaction.org/2012/11/15/what-the-frack-drill-rig-goes-pinkwashing-for-breast-cancer/

Breast Cancer Action. (2014d). Fracking and its connection to breast cancer. *Webinar.* http://bcaction.org/resources/webinars/fracking-and-its-connection-to-breast-cancer/

Breast Cancer Fund. (2010). *State of the evidence: The connection between breast cancer and the environment by Janet Gray, Ph.D.* Retrieved from March 2, 2015, from http://www.breastcancerfund.org/assets/pdfs/publications/state-of-the-evidence-2010.pdf.

Breast Cancer Fund. (2014). *Support full disclosure of fracking chemicals.* https://secure3.convio.net/bcf/site/Advocacy?cmd=display&page=User Action&id=241

Brendtro, M. J. (1998). Breast cancer: Agenda setting through activism. *Advanced Practice Nursing Quarterly, 4*(1), 54–63.

Brenner, B. (2012). Interview by Zaylia A. Pluss in San Francisco, CA. Accessed through Sophia Smith Collection, Smith College 2012.

Brenner, B. (2002). *Exercise your mind,* Breast Cancer Action, Newsletter 58, March/April, 2000, http://www.bcaction.org/Pages/Searchable Pages/2000Newsletters/Newsletter058B.html

Brody, J. G., Tickner, J., & Rudel, R. A. (2005). Community initiated breast cancer and environment studies and the precautionary principle. *Environmental Health Perspectives, 113*, 920–925.

Brown, P. (2007). *Toxic exposures.* New York: Columbia University Press.

Brown, P., Zavestoski, S. M., McCormick, S., Mandelbaum, J., & Luebke, T. (2001). Print media coverage of environmental causation of breast cancer. *Sociology of Health & Illness, 23*, 747–752.

Brown, P., & Zayetoski, S. (2005). *Social movements in health.* Malden, MA: Blackwell.

Brown, P., Zavestoski, S., McCormick, S., Mayer, B., Morello-Frosch, R., & Altman, R. G. (2004). Embodied health movements: New approaches to social movements in health. *Sociology of Health & Illness, 26*(1), 50–80.

Bullard, R. D., & Johnson, G. S. (2000). Environmental justice: Grassroots activism and its impact on public policy decision-making. *Journal of Social Issues, 56*, 555–578.

Bullard, R. (1990). *Dumping in Dixie: Race, class, and environmental quality.* Boulder, CO: Westview.

Carson, R. (1994). *Silent spring: With an introduction by Al Gore.* Boston, MA: Houghton.

Cassamayo, M. (2001). *The politics of breast cancer.* Washington, DC: Georgetown University Press.

Committee on Energy & Commerce, Democrats. (2011). *Committee democrats release new report detailing hydraulic fracturing products.* http://democrats.energycommerce.house.gov/index.php?q=news/committee-democrats-release-new-report-detailing-hydraulic-fracturing-products

Creswell, J. (2009). *Research design: Qualitative, quantitative and mixed methods.* Thousand Oaks, CA: Sage.

Earp, J., French, E., & Gilke, M. (2008). *Patient advocacy for health care quality.* Sudbury, MA: Jones and Bartlett Publishers.

Ehrenreich, B. (2001). Welcome to cancerland: A mammogram leads to a cult of pink kitsch. *Harper's Magazine,* 47.

Eisenstein, Z. (2001). *Manmade breast cancer.* Ithaca, NY: Cornell University Press.

Elliott, C. (2007). Pink!: Community, contestation, and the color of breast cancer. *Canadian Journal of Communication, 32,* 521–536.

Environmental Protection Agency. (2014a). *Natural gas extraction-hydraulic fracturing.* http://www2.epa.gov/hydraulicfracturing

Environmental Protection Agency. (2014b). *Endocrine disruptor research initiative, fact sheet.* http://www.epa.gov/edrlupvx/edrifact.html

Environmental Protection Agency. (2012a). *Benzene.* http://www.epa.gov/ttn/atw/hlthef/benzene.html

Environmental Protection Agency. (2012b). *Toluene.* http://www.epa.gov/ttn/atw/hlthef/toluene.html

Environmental Working Group. (2009). *Pollution in minority newborns: BPA and other cord blood pollutants.* Retrieved from www.ewg.org

Food and Water Watch. (2013). *The social costs of fracking.* http://documents.foodandwaterwatch.org/doc/Social_Costs_of_Fracking.pdf

Ford. *Calling all warriors.* May 17, 2007, from http://www.fordvehicles.com/warriorsinpink/wip/

Gerber, E. (1999). *The populist paradox: Interest group influence and the promise of direct legislation.* Princeton, NJ: Princeton University Press.

Goffman, E. (1974). *Frame analysis: An essay on the organization of experience.* New York: Harper & Row.

Heaney, M., & McClurg, S. (2009). Social networks and American politics: Introduction to the special issue. *American Politics Research, 37,* 727.

Hughes, B. (2015). *Baker Hughes Supports Susan G. Komen's mission to end breast cancer forever.* http://public.bakerhughes.com/pink/ (Accessed March 30, 2015).

Institute of Medicine. (2011). *Breast cancer and the environment: A life course approach* [Online]. http://www.iom.edu/Reports/2011/Breast-Cancer-and-the-Environment-A-Life-Course-Approach.aspx (Accessed June 2011)

Institute of Medicine. (2011). *IOM report identifies steps that may reduce women's risk for breast cancer associated with environmental factors.* http://www.iom.edu/Reports/2011/Breast-Cancer-and-the-Environment-A-Life-Course-Approach/Press-Release.aspx

Institute of Medicine. (1999). *Toward environmental justice: Research, education, and health policy needs.* Washington, DC: National Academy Press.

Kasper, A. S., & Ferguson, S. (2000). *Breast cancer.* New York: Palgrave Macmillan.

Kedrowski, K., & Sarow, M. S. (2007). *Cancer activism.* Chicago: University of Illinois Press.

King, S. (2008). *Pink Ribbons, Inc.: Breast cancer and the politics of philanthropy.* Minneapolis: University of Minnesota Press.

King, S. (2004). Pink Ribbons, Inc.: Breast cancer activism and the politics of philanthropy. *International Journal of Qualitative Studies in Education (QSE), 17,* 473–492.

Klawiter, M. (2008). *The biopolitics of breast cancer.* Minneapolis: University of Minnesota Press.

Knoke, D., & Yang, S. (2008). *Social network analysis.* Thousand Oaks, CA: Sage.

Kolker, E. S. (2004). Framing as a cultural resource in health social movements: Funding activism and the breast cancer movement in the US 1990–1993. *Sociology of Health & Illness, 26,* 820–844.

Komen Foundation. (2012). Massachusetts. *About Us.* http://www.komen mass.org/site/c.6oIEJTPxGcISF/b.8708397/k.C987/About_Us.htm

Komen Foundation. (2011, October 22). *Susan G. Komen for the Cure BPA Statement.* https://ww5.komen.org/uploadedFiles/Content_Binaries/BPAStatementOctober2011.pdf

Komen Foundation. (2011). *You Can Do This.* Promotional Materials sent in the mail.

Komen Foundation. (2010). *Circle of promise campaign.* Retrieved from http://www.komen.org

Komen Foundation. (2007). We're looking for some women to work around the house. *Organizational material.*

Komen Foundation. *How funds are used.* November 30, 2006, from http://www.komen.org/intradoc-cgi/idc_cgi_isapi.dll?IdcService=SS_GET _PAGE&nodeId=525

Komen Foundation. (2010). *What are your concerns and priorities concerning environmental risk factors for breast cancer?* Email sent out to members.

Komen Foundation. (2009). *Advocacy Alliance.* http://ww5.komen.org/GetInvolved/kaa.html

Kushner, R. (1982). *Why me? What every woman should know about breast cancer.* New York: Henry Holt & Co.

Leopold, E. (1999). *A darker ribbon: Breast cancer, women, and their doctors in the twentieth century.* Boston, MA: Beacon Press.

Lerner, B. (2001). *Breast cancer wars.* London, UK: Oxford University Press.

Lerner, B. H. (2002b). TIMELINE: Breast cancer activism: Past lessons, future directions. *Nature Reviews Cancer, 2,* 225–229.

Ley, B. L. (2009). *From pink to green.* New Brunswick, NJ: Rutgers University Press.

Lorde, A. (2006). *The cancer journals.* Special edition. San Francisco: Aunt Lute Books.

Lupton, D. (1994). The body in medicine. In *Medicine as culture. Illness disease and the body in western society.* London: Sage Publications.

Martin, E. (1999). The egg and the sperm: How science has constructed a romance based on stereotypical male-female roles. In J. Price & M. Shildrick (Eds.), *Feminist theory and the body: A reader* (pp. 179–189). New York: Routledge.

Martin, E. (1998). The fetus as intruder. In R. Davis-Floyd & J. Dumit (Eds.), *Cyborg babies*. New York: Routledge.

Massachusetts Breast Cancer Coalition. (2015). www.mbcc.org

Mayer, M. (1998). *Advanced breast cancer: A guide to living with metastatic disease*. Beijing: O'Reilly Media Inc.

McAdam, D. (1988). *Freedom summer*. New York: Oxford University Press.

McClintock, A. (1996). No longer in a future heaven: Nationalism, gender, and race. In G. Eley & R. G. Suny (Eds.), *Becoming national: A reader* (pp. 260–285). New York: Oxford University Press.

McCormick, S. (2009). *Mobilizing science*. Philadelphia, PA: Temple University Press.

McCormick, S. (2010). *No family history*. Lanham, MD: Rowman and Littlefield.

McDermott-Levy, R., Kaktins, N., & Sattler, B. (2013). Fracking, the environment, and health: New energy practices may threaten public health. *American Journal of Nursing, 113*(6), 45–51.

Meyer, D. S., & Whittier, N. (1994). Social movement spillover. *Social Problems, 41*, 277–298.

Miles, M., & Huberman, M. (Eds.). (1994). *Qualitative data analysis*. Thousand Oaks, CA: Sage.

Mitchell, J. C. (1969). The concept and use of social networks. In J. C. Mitchell (Ed.), *Social networks in urban situations*. Manchester, England: Manchester University Press.

Montini, T., & Ruzek, S. (1989). Overturning orthodoxy: The emergence of breast cancer treatment policy. *Research in Sociology of Health Care, 8*, 3–32.

National Breast Cancer Awareness Month. November 30, 2006, from http://www.whitehouse.gov/news/releases/2005/09/20050930-10.html

National Breast Cancer Coalition. (2011–2012). Organizational materials.

National Cancer Institute. *2005 Fact book*. http://fmb.cancer.gov/financial/attachments/FY-2005-FACT-BOOK-FINAL.pdf.

National Cancer Institute. (2008–2009). *Environmental factors in cancer*. Washington, DC: President's Cancer Panel, National Cancer Institute [Online]. http://deainfo.nci.nih.gov/advisory/pcp/annualReports/index.htm (Accessed January 6, 2013).

National Cancer Institute. (2010). Retrieved from www.nci.org

National Cancer Institute. (2008). *Questions and answers about the breast cancer and the environment on long island study*. Retrieved March 2, 2015, from http://www.cancer.gov/newscenter/qa/2002/long-island-environmentqa.

Neuman, W. L. (2006). *Social research methods* (6th ed.). Boston, MA: University of Wisconsin at Whitewater.

Parthasarathy, S. (2010). Breaking the expertise barrier: Understanding activist strategies in science and technology policy domains. *Science and Public Policy, 37*, 355–367.

Patel, K., & Rushefsky, M. (2005). *The politics of public health in the United States.* Armank, NY: M.E. Sharpe.

Pezzullo, P. C. (2003). Resisting "national breast cancer awareness month": The rhetoric of counterpublics and their cultural performances. *Quarterly Journal of Speech, 89*, 345–365.

Potts, L. K. (2004a). An epidemiology of women's lives: The environmental risk of breast cancer. *Critical Public Health, 14*(2), 133–147.

Potts, L. (2004b). Mapping citizen expertise about environmental risk of breast cancer. *Critical Social Policy, 24*, 550–574.

Potts, L. K. (2000). *Ideologies of breast cancer: Feminist perspectives.* New York, NY: Palgrave Macmillan.

Prakash, A., & Gugerty, M. K. (Eds.). (2010). *Advocacy organizations and collective action.* New York: Cambridge University Press.

Sedgwick, E. K. (1999). Breast cancer: An adventure in applied deconstruction. In J. Price & M. Schildrick (Eds.), *Feminist theory and the body: A reader.* New York: Routledge, 153–156.

Schonfelder, G., Wittoht, W., Hopp, H., Talsness, C. E., Paul, M., & Chahoud, I. (2002). Parent bisphenol A accumulation in the human maternal-fetal-placental unit. *Environmental Health Perspective, 110* (11), A703–A707.

Silent Spring Institute. (2015). *Body burden.* www.http://www.silentspring.org/body-burden (Accessed February 28, 2015).

Snow, D., & Benford, R. (1988). Ideology, frame resonance, and participant mobilization. *International Social Movement Research, 1*, 197–217.

Snow, D., Rochford, E. B., Worden, S. K., & Benford, R. D. (1986). Frame alignment processes, micromobilization, and movement participation. *American Sociological Review, 51*, 464–481.

Sontag, S. (2001). *Illness as metaphor.* New York: Picador.

Stacey, J. (1997). *Teratologies: A cultural study of cancer.* London: Routledge.

Stein, R. (2004). *New perspectives on environmental justice.* New Brunswick, NJ: Rutgers University Press.

Steingraber, S. (1997a). Mechanisms, proof, and unmet needs: The perspective of a cancer activist. *Environmental Health Perspectives, 105*, 685–687.

Steingraber, S. (1997b). *Living down stream.* Reading, MA: Wesley.

Strolovich, D. Z. (2007). *Affirmative advocacy: Race, class, and gender in interest group politics.* Chicago, IL: University of Chicago Press.

Sulik, G. (2012). *Pink Ribbon Blues: How breast cancer culture undermines women's health.* Oxford: Oxford University Press.

Swissler, M. (2003). Compromised? The Susan G. Komen Foundation is tied up in private interests that run counter to its mission. *Creative Loafing, 17*, 30–39.

Swissler, M. A. (2002). *The marketing of breast cancer*. Retrieved from AlterNet.org

Turshen, M. (2007). *Women's health movements: A global force for change*. New York: Palgrave Macmillan.

Wailoo, K. (2011). *How cancer crossed the color line*. Oxford: Oxford University Press.

Weisman, C. S. (2000). Breast cancer policymaking. In A. S. Kasper & J. S. Ferguson (Eds.), *Breast cancer: Society shapes an epidemic* (pp. 213–244). New York: St. Martin's Press.

World Health Organization. (2008, June 29). *Cancer*. http://www.who.int/mediacentre/factsheets/fs297/en/index.html

World Health Organization. (2008, June 29). *Screening for breast cancer*. http://www.who.int/cancer/detection/breastcancer/en/

Young, M. (2010). The Price of advocacy: Mobilization and maintenance in advocacy organizations. In A. Prakash & M. K. Gugerty (Eds.), *Advocacy organizations and collective action* (pp. 31–57). New York: Cambridge University Press.

Index

About the Author

KRISTEN ABATSIS MCHENRY, PhD, is a faculty member at the University of Massachusetts, Dartmouth, in the Women's and Gender Studies Department. She earned her doctorate in political science from the University of Massachusetts Amherst, where her dissertation research was on breast cancer advocacy. She also holds an MA in women's and gender studies from Georgia State University. Her research interests include women's health, environment, and breast cancer advocacy. Her publications include topics related to women's health, environment, and social movement organizations. Her next research project covers the links between breast cancer, fracking, and environmental health.